The Ultimate
Creatine
Handbook

The Ultimate
CREATINE
Handbook

THE SAFE ALTERNATIVE FOR
HEALTHY MUSCLE BUILDING

Dr. Joseph A. Debé & Donna Caruso

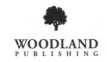

WOODLAND
PUBLISHING

The CIP record for this book is available from the Library of Congress.

For ordering information, contact:
Woodland Publishing
448 East 800 North, Orem, Utah 84097
(800) 777-2665

Note: The information in this book is for educational purposes only and is not recommended as a means of diagnosing or treating an illness. All matters concerning physical and mental health should be supervised by a health practitioner knowledgeable in treating that particular condition. Neither the publisher nor author directly or indirectly dispenses medical advice, nor do they prescribe any remedies or assume any responsibility for those who choose to treat themselves.

ISBN 1-58054-355-3

Printed in the United States of America

Please visit our website:
www.woodlandpublishing.com

To my favorite daughter, Danielle
J.A.D.

———————————————

Donna Caruso dedicates this book to Philip, an
enthusiastic athlete and a true friend

Acknowledgments

Thanks to my coauthor, Donna Caruso, for being such a joy to work with and for putting up with my many revisions to the book.

I would like to thank Oscar Ramjeet, president of Nature's Value, Inc., for his patience in dealing with my barrage of phone calls and questions about creatine source material. Oscar's "behind-the-scenes" knowledge of nutritional supplement manufacturing was invaluable to the creation of this book.

Thanks to my wife, Jennifer, for her typical whole-hearted support and understanding during my involvement in this lengthy project.

Finally, I would like to pay tribute to the forward-thinkers who discovered the value of supplemental creatine and all the brilliant researchers who continue to expand our knowledge of the many ways that creatine can improve our lives. Without them, this book would not exist.

Joseph A. Debé, DC, DACBN, CCN

Contents

Creatine: An Introduction

WHEN IT COMES to nutritional supplements that build strength and muscle, nothing can touch creatine. It is the most studied and most widely used sports supplement of all time. And what's even better is that from everything we know, it's also remarkably safe.

Creatine has been used by many popular sports figures, most notably baseball's home-run sluggers Barry Bonds and Mark McGwire. In fact, creatine is used by a large percentage of athletes in various Olympic competitions, and in many professional sports, such as football and baseball.

Furthermore, all the research about creatine has shown it is not only effective for many different types of sports and exercise, it is also helpful for many health problems and could also be useful to prevent these problems from developing in the first place. Today, ongoing research may find additional uses for creatine supplementation for people suffering from various conditions including Parkinson's disease, muscular dystrophy, and some of the signs of aging.

But even though creatine is well-studied and appears to have no serious side effects, it still isn't a good idea to just walk into a health food store, buy some and take it. In order for creatine to work and for you to protect your health and well-being, you must first know what you are doing. You need to know:

- Which types of sports and exercise benefit from creatine use and which do not.
- Which health factors and conditions may improve with creatine supplementation.
- Why all creatine products are not the same and how you can find the one that's right for you.
- How to take creatine for maximum benefit.
- Which forms of creatine are the most effective and the best value for your money.
- What possible side effects can occur with creatine use.
- Who should NOT use creatine and why.
- Why some people should have medical supervision for creatine supplementation.
- How creatine is different from other muscle-building supplements such as "andro" (androstenedione) or steroids.
- How to start taking creatine and whether or not you should begin by loading (taking higher amounts initially).
- Whether it is a good idea to cycle creatine (take it for certain periods of time and then stop for a while).
- Whether you really need creatine to perform at your best and compete with others in your sport.

If you are already taking creatine and are not certain if you're doing it the right way or to your best advantage, if you have friends using creatine and wonder if you will get the same results, or if you're just interested in learning more about creatine before deciding whether to try it, this book is for you.

In this book, you will learn everything you need to know about creatine from Dr. Joseph Debé, a sports chiropractor, board certified nutritionist and former competitive weight lifter who has used creatine himself. Over the years, Dr. Debé has also treated national and world-champion athletes, monitoring their use of creatine to improve athletic performance. As you will see, he is a strong believer in creatine because he has seen that it works. Dr. Debé will explain to you:

• Why creatine is such a popular supplement
• What creatine is and where it is found in the body
• How creatine works to build muscle
• The history of creatine use as a muscle-building supplement
• How creatine can benefit your health
• How creatine enhances sports performance
• How to buy the right creatine product
• How to use creatine for maximum benefits
• Problems associated with creatine use
• The benefits of other muscle-building supplements
• How to create your own program for better health and sports performance

By the time you finish reading this book, you will know whether or not creatine is right for you, how to put it to use, and what results you can realistically expect.

So whether you're a "weekend warrior," a professional football player, a bodybuilder, an older man or woman trying to build up strength, or just someone who wants to feel better and perform to the maximum in your sport, creatine may well provide the boost you are seeking.

CHAPTER ONE

A Creatine Overview

THIS CHAPTER WILL profile creatine and its uses, touching on the major issues discussed in greater detail later in this book.

Q: Why is creatine the most popular sports supplement today?
A: Because it really works. Out of all the sports supplements available, creatine is the one with the greatest amount of research. To date, there are hundreds of studies on creatine and more than 70 percent of these studies have found it to be of benefit to athletes wanting to build muscle and strength.

Q: What does creatine actually do, and how do people know that it really works?
A: Creatine increases energy production for muscular contraction, which has the end result of increasing strength and power output for short-term intense athletic activities. It also increases muscle mass. We know it does these things and actually works because of the many studies published in recognized scientific

journals and because we can actually see the results in ourselves and in people we know who use creatine.

Q: *Have you seen these results with people you know or with yourself?*
A: Yes, I have. Creatine has worked well for me and for many of the people I've worked with and known over the years.

Q: *What are the major benefits people can obtain from using creatine supplements?*
A: Creatine increases power output and the ability to exert force. These translate into greater strength for weight lifters, faster sprinting for runners, and better workouts for athletes engaging in weight training and short-term high-intensity exercise routines, quicker recovery from exercise, and increased muscle mass for most of those using it.

Q: *Aside from athletes and bodybuilders, how do others benefit from greater strength and more muscle?*
A: Increased strength and muscle mass are vastly underestimated factors in health and wellness. For example, a thirty-year study found that individuals with the greatest grip strength have the lowest overall risk of death.

Better strength and muscle mean a better physical appearance for both men and women (including women who want to lose weight), better mood, stronger bones, lowered risk of diabetes, improvement in the symptoms of arthritis and fibromyalgia, increased energy levels, and greater ease in carrying out everyday activities, along with a lowered risk of injury. Loss of muscle mass is associated with weakened immunity, declining health in general, and the aging process. So greater strength and muscle mass are highly beneficial for everyone.

Q: What are some of creatine's health benefits?
A: Research on creatine has shown that it may help people with neuro-degenerative disorders, muscular dystrophies, and congestive heart failure, as well as certain signs of the aging process. Creatine has also been shown to improve rehabilitation from musculoskeletal injuries, and there is evidence that it may be beneficial for some conditions related to insulin resistance. Elevated blood cholesterol and triglyceride levels also improve with creatine supplementation. Overall, these health studies on creatine have a lot of important implications for many different disorders (see Chapter Five).

Q: Who actually uses creatine?
A: Many professional athletes use creatine, as do many athletes in Olympic, collegiate, and high school sports. Several studies have surveyed high school athletes to determine how many are using creatine and the results range from a low of about 5.6 percent to a high of about 30 percent, depending on the sport and locale.

The high figure of 30 percent was for a group of football players, who are the most likely to use creatine. Studies have found that both male and female athletes use creatine, and they are of all ages and in almost every sport. It's especially popular with bodybuilders and individuals who want to improve their physical appearance (a major reason for use found among high school athletes). As I will explain later, I do not recommend creatine for younger athletes, but the fact is that many are using it (see Chapter Nine).

Q: So not everyone using creatine is involved in sports?
A: That's right. In addition to people who want to improve their bodies, there are medical patients who are given creatine by their doctors to help with various health problems, including

neuromuscular conditions and heart failure, as we've already mentioned.

Q: *What are the approximate annual sales for creatine?*
A: In 1999, annual sales of creatine in this country were estimated at about $400 million and use appears to have grown since that time. So it's a very popular, widely used supplement.

Q: *You said that people in many different sports use creatine. But isn't it true that creatine does not help with every sport?*
A: That's correct. Many people, especially young athletes, don't know a lot about creatine and believe it will help their sports performance, but in quite a few ~~es~~ they're wrong. Creatine's main benefits are for sports and exercise that involve short-term bursts of energy, like football and weight lifting. Creatine is not that effective for sports involving long-term endurance, such as marathon running—it can even be a hindrance (see Chapter Six).

Q: *Do you believe that creatine actually makes a difference in athletic performance? In the sports and activities where it helps, do you see a difference between people who are using creatine and people who are not?*
A: Yes. You can see a difference. But as I explained, you will only see it in a sport where there is an emphasis on quick power production or in people who want to increase muscle mass. And you have to remember that creatine will not work the same way in everyone. The effect varies from individual to individual for various reasons, including genetic factors and diet. Creatine does not work for everyone, but it certainly does work for a lot of people. And it does make a difference.

Q: *We keep hearing that creatine is safe and that no one has ever*

suggested that it be monitored or banned. But why is it safer than other muscle-building supplements, like andro or steroids?
A: Creatine is very safe and that has been proven over many years with hundreds of studies and the millions of people who have used it. Creatine is a very different substance from andro or steroids, as you will see later on (Chapters Six and Ten).

Creatine's main action is to increase energy production in the cells. Steroids, on the other hand, influence messaging between different tissues in the body, and steroid hormones can be converted into other hormones and upset the balance of the endocrine system. That can have some very negative health effects, including liver and heart damage and possible links to cancer.

In short, there are a lot of published studies showing dangerous side effects with andro and steroids, but creatine studies consistently show no adverse side effects. So while anabolic steroids can build muscle, they do so in a different way and only creatine has been proven to be safe.

Q: *Should people using creatine be under a doctor's supervision, rather than just going to the health food store, buying it, and taking it on their own?*
A: For most people, continual medical supervision is not necessary. But as you will see later on (Chapter Nine), there are some people who need to see a physician first because creatine could potentially be dangerous for them if they have certain medical conditions, including kidney disorders, or are taking certain medications.

In addition, there are no studies proving that creatine is safe for people under the age of 18, so anyone younger than 18 should definitely consult a qualified physician or other health care professional before using it. Just make sure your doctor is familiar with creatine and understands what it is and how it works.

Ron: From Super Strong to World Record-Holder

A longtime friend and patient, Ron Walsh was already a very strong power lifter when I met him a number of years ago. Ron had never used anabolic steroids or any other drugs, but he had experimented with a variety of natural supplements that were supposed to boost strength. If he found they didn't work, he stopped using them.

After reading the early reports about creatine, I suggested to Ron that he might want to give it a try. I instructed him on loading with creatine and then using a maintenance dose, but Ron preferred to use creatine his way. Believing that "if a little is good, a whole lot is better," Ron explained that he didn't have the time to mix up a creatine drink four times a day. So he put two tablespoons of creatine powder into his mouth, held it under his tongue for a while and then washed it down with water. He did this twice a day for the first week. And even though he knew the recommended dose was about 20 grams a day, Ron was taking about 40 to 60 grams a day.

Following the first week, Ron reduced his dose to just one a day instead of two. He told me that right after the loading phase, he saw an immediate improvement, feeling tighter and stronger. But he also had some negative side effects, like cramps and intestinal gas, so he reduced the dose to 1 tablespoon a day, (about 10 grams of creatine), adding another tablespoon twenty minutes before workouts.

Ron used creatine for four years, until he retired from power lifting. He would cycle it three to four months on and one month off. Before meets, Ron always took a mouthful of creatine (about 4 tablespoons).

While he was using creatine, Ron would typically gain 10 to 12 pounds in four to six weeks, and he said his body felt harder and he was more energetic and confident. He also reported having fewer injuries to his joints and connective tissues.

Ron observed that using creatine appeared to cause everything to swell and get bigger, including his neck and fingers. His face would flush and when he dead lifted maximum weights, he felt increased nasal pressure, and his eyes would tear. Ron believes that his blood pressure also increased while he was using creatine.

Creatine is also responsible for Ron having to pay an increased life insurance premium because when he started using creatine, his blood creatinine levels became elevated, which is commonly interpreted as a sign of kidney failure. In Ron's case, however, the elevated creatinine was due to his creatine supplements. As we'll later discuss, creatine is converted to creatinine in the muscle, transported through the blood to the kidneys, and excreted in the urine.

Ron believes that creatine helped him to become a national champion. He won both the International Power Lifting Association National Championship and the American Drug-Free Powerlifting Association Lifetime Drug-Free National Championship. Creatine also helped Ron to successfully compete against other lifters in the American Power Lifting Federation and the International Power Lifting Federation, many of whom were using performance-enhancing drugs.

Competing in the 242-pound weight class, Ron has officially dead lifted 700 pounds and has set world records in the IPA Amateur (Drug-Free) Division with a squat of 720 pounds and a bench press of 551 pounds.

How did Ron know that creatine was really helping him? As an example, when he was not taking creatine in August 1996, Ron missed a 575 pound bench press. Then, after using creatine for six weeks, he was able to bench press 575 pounds twice.

In addition, Ron observed that while he was not using creatine for about a month, he was smaller, less tight, less energetic and strong, and found power lifting less enjoyable.

As for the side effects Ron experienced, he is very in tune with his body, and there could be a connection between some of them and creatine, even though no scientific study has found a direct correlation. However, Ron took about twenty different natural supplements on a regular basis, and it is likely that some of the adverse reactions he experienced were actually due to something else. Most notably, Ron took high doses of ephedra-containing supplements, which are known to elevate blood pressure. Still, we can't totally exonerate creatine as the cause of some of his symptoms.

It is possible that Ron reacted to creatine in a way that most people would not or that the higher doses he was using may have had a role in causing these side effects. It is always safer to use creatine at the recommended dose.

Q: *Are there any dangers from using creatine, such as unwanted side effects?*
A: Other than weight gain (in the form of muscle), studies have not shown any proof of adverse side effects. Even though studies have found supplemental creatine to be free of side effects other than weight gain, I believe a given individual may react adversely to any compound. Individual reactions to any supplement, or food for that matter, is a distinct possibility, so creatine could possibly cause side effects in a small number of sensitive people.

Q: *What do people need to know before deciding whether or not to use creatine?*
A: They should know how it works in the body and what effects it produces. Creatine is not going to help in every sport. It is beneficial for strength athletes but not so much for endurance athletes, so people need to know if creatine will produce the specific benefits they are looking for. They also need to know how to take it, how much to take, what it costs, and what possible side effects to watch out for.

Q: *What about using creatine for anti-aging? Can it be helpful?*
A: Yes, I think it can. I am actually very excited about creatine's possible applications for anti-aging. With aging, there is a loss of muscle mass, which is probably the single most important change in the body. If you can build muscle as you're aging, you will be healthier, you will probably live longer and you will have a better quality of life. In studies of older people, creatine has been found to increase strength and muscle mass. So creatine can be a great anti-aging supplement, especially if you combine it with exercise.

Creatine also appears to benefit mental function and protect against development of neuro-degenerative diseases. Additionally, creatine supplementation produces a variety of beneficial physiological effects, such as improved circulation. We will talk more about creatine's anti-aging properties later on in this book (Chapter Eleven).

Q: *What is your personal opinion about creatine?*
A: I think it's a valuable supplement—a great sports supplement. Creatine is the best available supplement for increasing strength, and nothing works as quickly or as well. For decades, people have been looking for a natural compound that could produce a measurable effect on muscle building, but there wasn't anything that had a dramatic effect. People turned to anabolic steroids to try to get better results, but they turned out to be very danger-ous and undesirable.

Then creatine came along. Now, by using creatine, people can build muscle and increase strength in a safe way. It works very quickly and very consistently, especially when accompanied by a regular exercise or training program. I also think it is an impor-tant supplement for the different medical conditions we men-tioned. And I believe that more medical applications, including those of anti-aging, will be found in the future.

Q: *You said that you used creatine yourself. How well did it work for you?*
A: I used creatine toward the end of my weight lifting career, at a time when creatine supplements were just becoming popular. I never used it in competition, but only used it for weight training.

I definitely noticed a rapid effect and a lot of my patients have also noticed that within a day or two of supplementing, there is a noticeable increase in strength. I find that there can be a 10 percent or greater improvement in the number of repetitions you can do. There is also an increase in body weight—which in some cases, can be a detriment, such as when it pushes you up to the next weight class, so you have to monitor your results very carefully. This weight gain is in muscle mass, with no increase in body fat. A few studies have actually found creatine to reduce body fat percentage.

As for side effects, I've had a little bit of cramping during exercise, but only during the actual set of exercise, and nothing that was too troubling. (Actually, it's difficult to say if the cramping was caused by the creatine because I have also experienced muscle cramps when not using creatine.) I've used creatine at a few different times over the years. Most recently, after supplementing with creatine for a couple of weeks, I gained six pounds and my musculature looked about five years younger—bigger, more solid and more vascular. I also felt more energetic and had a greater sense of mental-emotional well-being. I've used it with a loading phase a couple of times and I've also used it at a low dose on a daily basis, and I've seen results both ways, with increased strength and greater muscle mass. Overall, I think it's a pretty impressive supplement.

Points to Remember

- Creatine is the strength and muscle-building supplement with the greatest amount of research, having been the subject of hundreds of studies.
- Creatine boosts energy production for muscular contraction, which increases strength and power output for short-term intense athletic activities. It also speeds recovery after exertion.
- Creatine benefits athletes in various sports, such as providing greater strength for weight lifters, faster sprinting for runners, and better workouts for those using weight training.
- Creatine also has benefits for people with certain medical conditions, including neuromuscular disorders such as muscular dystrophy, congestive heart failure and certain aspects of aging.
- Many professional athletes use creatine, as do non-professional athletes, including college and high school students.
- Creatine helps in activities requiring short-term bursts of energy but is not generally helpful in endurance activities.
- Although most people benefit, the effects of creatine vary among individuals and it may not work for everyone.
- Creatine studies show no serious side effects, unlike many other supplements such as andro and steroids.
- It's a good idea to check with your health care professional before using creatine to be certain you don't have any medical conditions or are not taking any medications that might make creatine unsafe for you.
- It's important to know about creatine before you use it, so you will be certain that it's right for you. You will also have the knowledge to use it for maximum effect.

CHAPTER TWO

What Is Creatine and What Is Its Role in Creating Energy?

IN THIS CHAPTER, you will learn all about creatine—what it is, where it is found naturally in the body, how our bodies make it, how much is in the average person's body, good dietary sources, and why many people choose to use creatine supplements. You will also find out how your body creates energy, what happens when creatine levels are low, and how creatine supplements can benefit athletic performance.

Q: Exactly what is creatine?
A: Creatine is a naturally occurring compound in the human body that is made from three amino acids: arginine, glycine, and methionine. The scientific name for creatine is N-methyl-guanidinoacetic acid. Although technically an amino acid itself, creatine is more properly a nutrient that is made up of these three amino acids.

Q: What are amino acids and why are they important?
A: Amino acids are molecules that are the building blocks of pro-

tein, which is the main compound that forms the structures or the tissues of the body. Amino acids have many functions, including neurotransmitter action involving brain function, detoxification of various compounds and transportation of minerals throughout the body.

There are twenty-two amino acids in the protein structure of human beings, eight of them classified as essential, several semi-essential, and the rest non-essential. Essential amino acids are the ones that the body can't manufacture and that have to be obtained from the diet. Semi-essential amino acids can be made from essential amino acids, but there are often not enough to meet the body's needs, so some of these amino acids have to be supplied by the diet. And non-essential amino acids are the ones that the body can manufacture freely and are not normally needed in the diet. For various reasons, however, individuals can also be deficient in the non-essential amino acids.

Q: How does the body make creatine?
A: Creatine is made from arginine, glycine, and methionine. These amino acids are extracted from the food we eat, and arginine and glycine can also be manufactured in the body.

Q: Why are these three amino acids important?
A: In addition to creatine synthesis, these amino acids have many other important roles in human physiology. Arginine is a semi-essential amino acid that aids ammonia detoxification, stimulates the release of insulin and growth hormone and helps injuries to heal. As a precursor to nitric oxide, arginine also influences immune system function and blood vessel health.

Glycine is a non-essential amino acid that is a component of many proteins, helps in detoxification, can be useful in treating certain types of schizophrenia, and also stimulates the release of growth hormone. As a component of bile acids, glycine also plays a role in cholesterol excretion and in the absorption of fatty acids and fat soluble nutrients.

Methionine is an essential amino acid that helps to make hormones more active, assists in detoxification and regulates some genetic processes. It also plays a role in protection against cancer formation and, as a source of sulfur, is important for joint and connective tissue health. These are a few of the known functions of these amino acids.

Q: *Where is creatine made in the body?*
A: It is made primarily in the liver, kidneys, and pancreas.

Q: *And where is it found in the body?*
A: Once it is absorbed from our food or synthesized in the body, creatine is transported by the circulatory system to the muscle cells, where creatine transporters shuttle it into these cells. So almost all of the body's creatine, an estimated 95 percent, is found in the muscles. Smaller amounts are found in other tissues, including the liver, brain, kidneys, heart, smooth muscles, endothelial cells, macrophages (a type of white blood cell) and testes.

Inside muscle cells, about two-thirds of the creatine becomes bound to a phosphate group and is referred to as creatine phosphate. The remaining creatine is free or plain creatine. It is the creatine phosphate that is the energy-producing form.

Q: *Does everyone have creatine in their bodies at all times?*
A: Yes, we all have some creatine in our bodies all the time, including the creatine that the body manufactures and the creatine that we get from certain foods that have high creatine contents.

Q: *How much total creatine is found in the average person's body?*

A: An average person weighs about 70 kilograms or 154 pounds and this individual would have an average of about 120 grams of creatine in the body at any given time. The body typically breaks down about 2 grams of creatine per day, which needs to be replaced. The body can manufacture some of what it needs, but the balance has to come from dietary sources.

Q: What are some of the best dietary sources of creatine?
A: The best sources of creatine are meat and fish. For instance, herring has about 3 grams per pound, pork about 2.3 grams per pound, beef and salmon about 2 grams per pound, and tuna about 1.8 grams per pound.

Q: What if you're a strict vegetarian and don't eat meat or fish?
A: Then your dietary intake of creatine would be less than the average person's. Your body would still be manufacturing creatine and all other things being equal, you could be very healthy, but without supplementation, you might not have the same physical strength as someone with a higher creatine intake.

Q: If we already have creatine in our bodies, why should we consider taking it as a supplement?
A: First of all, there are many reasons why the body might not have sufficient creatine. As we've just said, your diet may not be supplying adequate amounts. About half the creatine in the body is made internally, with the rest supplied from the food we eat. So anyone who is a strict vegetarian or who is not eating a diet with enough protein rich in creatine could be deficient in creatine.

Second, there can be genetic factors. There are at least three different genetic defects that have been identified as resulting in impaired metabolism due to inadequate creatine activity. So your genetic makeup might increase your need for supplemental creatine.

Mark: Creatine Is a Supplement

Mark, a 17-year-old football player, was about to go into his senior year of high school. Hoping to make the varsity team, Mark was worried because he was on the small side. He felt hopeful when his football coach told him that he could be a starting player if he gained 15 pounds and brought his power clean single repetition maximum to 185 pounds. But he was also worried. Mark had always had trouble gaining weight, and his power clean was only 170 pounds.

Wanting to help their son, Mark's parents took him to my office for a consultation. After taking his history and talking with Mark and his parents, I discovered that Mark's diet and exercise routine had a lot of room for improvement. His weight training wasn't consistent or intense enough. Mark was interested in using creatine because many of his friends were using it and getting good results.

I explained to Mark and his parents that creatine is a great supplement, but it is still only a supplement and when you use it, you also have to work on your diet, exercise, and rest, or it won't do its work.

Mark, his parents and I all agreed that Mark would follow a new diet and exercise routine for a month. If he wasn't making good progress after that time, we would then add creatine as a supplement.

After a month, Mark was surprised to find that he had put on five pounds of weight and had increased his power clean by ten pounds. Since he was making good progress, Mark decided to continue with this program and by the time football camp began, he had gained a total of 9 pounds. Mark's coach was impressed by his progress and decided to let Mark start, even though his body weight was still a bit low. The coach was also pleased with his increase in the power clean.

Because he has done so well with these changes, Mark has decided not to use creatine for now. Although he says he may use it in the future, Mark told me that he realizes that a proper diet and consistent hard work are the most important factors for improving sports performance.

Third, certain people are deficient in the amino acids needed to make creatine. These amino acids could be lacking as a result of a poor diet, maldigestion, malabsorption, or could be depleted as a result of different causes, including toxicity in the body, which can drain arginine, methionine, and glycine levels. Other nutrient deficiencies and biochemical imbalances can also result in low creatine status.

Q: Is there also a difference in creatine levels depending on the amount of each person's physical activity?
A: Yes, that is another important factor. People who are more physically active and who exercise regularly are going to use up more creatine, so they will have a greater need to replenish their stores than someone who is not so physically active.

Q: Can the body's stores of creatine run out and if so, what makes that happen?
A: Our creatine stores never run out, but the available form, creatine phosphate, can be rapidly depleted to a level that impairs energy production. In fact, after five to ten seconds of very intense activity, the body's creatine phosphate supply can be very low and can "run out" after only thirty seconds of such activity. It takes time for creatine phosphate stores to be replenished.

Q: Is there any way to get the body to make more creatine?
A: According to one published study, supplementing with arginine and glycine, two of the amino acids that comprise creatine, results in increased creatine synthesis in the body.

Q: Is the body limited in the amount of creatine it can produce?
A: Yes, and that's another reason why people may want to use supplements. When your body produces creatine, the creatine levels increase. At that point, production stops. So you can only

get to a certain level of creatine (about 120 total grams for an average person) through production inside the body.

However, when you take supplemental creatine, you can increase the levels of creatine within your cells to a much higher degree than you ever could just by having your body produce its optimum levels. So when you use supplemental creatine, you're really reaching a kind of supra-physiological level—you're getting levels of creatine into your cells that your body could never achieve on its own—up to about 125 percent of normal. Creatine phosphate levels may increase up to 140 percent of normal. Creatine supplementation literally makes us "super" men and women.

Q: *Exactly how does the body make energy?*
A: The body produces energy by breaking down food to release the energy in its chemical bonds, and it can also use its own tissues for energy by breaking them down.

Food is broken down into small molecules, which are transported into the mitochondria of the cells, which are the energy factories of the cells. Then there are a complex series of reactions called the Krebs cycle (or citric acid cycle), as the food components are converted into different compounds and go through a process called oxidative phosphorylation to produce an energy currency called ATP (adenosine triphosphate). The ATP ultimately produces energy by liberating a phosphate group and being converted into ADP (adenosine diphosphate) in the process. So when ATP is converted into ADP, energy is produced.

Here's where creatine comes in. Creatine phosphate donates its phosphate group to ADP, converting it back into ATP and thus increasing energy stores. In the process, creatine phosphate becomes free (inactive) creatine.

Q: When our internal creatine phosphate supplies run out, what does the body do to create more energy?

A: Creatine can be recharged. It can diffuse to the mitochondria where ATP donates a phosphate group to the creatine to regenerate creatine phosphate. Then we have more creatine phosphate to help with energy production.

But after very intense exercise lasting between 10 and 30 seconds, the body switches to another source of energy, another fuel system that's called anaerobic glycolysis. Glycolysis involves the breakdown of sugar or glucose to produce ATP. The problem is that the process also creates lactic acid, which creates muscle fatigue and pain during very intense exercise. In fact, lactic acid can even completely shut down muscle contraction.

So that is how the body compensates when creatine supplies run out. It switches to a different energy system, but one that has undesirable side effects.

Q: How does supplemental creatine help when the body has exhausted its own supplies?

A: Supplemental creatine increases creatine levels in the muscles and more importantly, increases the body's creatine phosphate levels. It is creatine phosphate, the energy-producing form of creatine, that makes up about two-thirds of the creatine inside our cells. So by increasing creatine phosphate, you have an enhanced source of energy.

Q: How does the creatine phosphate work?

A: One way of thinking about creatine phosphate is by comparing it to a battery recharger. If ATP is the battery, creatine phosphate is the recharger. When the battery starts to run down, the creatine phosphate restores energy levels, leading to more intense and prolonged muscle contraction.

Creatine also increases muscle cell size. It increases water retention within muscle cells and perhaps because of that, it also increases protein synthesis within muscle cells, causing the cells to become bigger and stronger. By doing these things, creatine gives us more stamina for short-term repetitive activities, delays fatigue and the onset of exhaustion, increases lean body mass and body weight (which can be a plus or minus, depending on the situation), shortens recovery time after exercise, and permits more power output for longer workouts.

Q: Is the supplemental creatine that we buy in the stores the same as the creatine in our bodies?
A: No. The creatine we buy is a synthetically manufactured product and not precisely the same. The major form we buy is creatine monohydrate, which is creatine with a water molecule attached to help with absorption. When creatine monohydrate is mixed with water, free creatine is formed.

Inside our cells are two types of creatine: free creatine, which is unbound creatine; and creatine phosphate, the active form of creatine, which is bound to a phosphate group.

When we take creatine supplements or eat foods with creatine in them, the creatine levels in the blood become elevated. Creatine is transported into our cells and some of it becomes bound to phosphate and becomes active.

Q: So taking creatine supplements can be helpful for people who are very active, even though we have other sources?
A: Yes. As you have seen, the body produces from 1 to 2 grams of creatine a day and the average person takes in from 1 to 2 grams a day from food. The average person also uses up 2 grams a day in physical activity. But people who regularly engage in sports and exercise, especially if they involve short bursts of intense energy, can easily get into a state of suboptimal creatine status. Taking a supplement can be very helpful for these active

people, giving them added energy and an ability to continue to play or work out without getting rapidly exhausted. Remember, supplemental creatine raises tissue concentrations way above normal.

Points to Remember

- Creatine is a naturally occurring compound in the body.
- Creatine is made from three amino acids: arginine, glycine, and methionine.
- The body makes from 1 to 2 grams of creatine a day, which is produced in the liver, kidneys, and pancreas.
- Ninety-five percent of the body's creatine is found in the muscles. Smaller amounts are in the liver, brain, kidneys, heart, smooth muscles, endothelial cells, macrophages and testes.
- The average person has about 120 grams of creatine in the body at any given time.
- Meat and fish are the best dietary sources of creatine.
- Many different factors can contribute to low levels of creatine in the body.
- The body's stores of creatine can run down very quickly, especially with very intense exercise.
- Supplemental creatine increases levels in the muscles and allows for more strength, stamina, and muscle growth, as well as delaying fatigue and increasing lean body mass and body weight.
- People who are physically active, especially those who engage in sports and exercise involving short bursts of intense activity, may require additional creatine.
- Supplemental creatine is a good way for many active people to increase their stamina, energy and physical strength.

CHAPTER THREE

How Does Creatine Work in The Body?

IN THIS CHAPTER, you will discover what goes on in your body to create energy, physical activity and muscular strength; what your muscles need in order to remain healthy and grow; what happens when your muscles are injured; and how creatine can have a positive effect on muscular strength and growth.

Q: What are the different muscles that make up the body and how do they function?
A: There are three basic classes of muscles: skeletal (or striated), smooth, and cardiac.

Q: Can you explain the role of skeletal muscles?
A: Skeletal muscles are the muscles attached to your bones, the ones you can see when you look at a person. For instance, if you look at an advanced bodybuilder, you can actually see the muscles showing through the skin. Those are the skeletal muscles. Skeletal muscle contraction is under our conscious control and that's why they are also called voluntary muscles.

Q: *What about smooth muscles?*
A: Smooth muscle contraction is normally not under our conscious control. These muscles operate without our having to consciously think about making them contract and are therefore called involuntary muscles. Smooth muscle is found in various organs in the body, such as the blood vessels, stomach, skin, and the intestinal tract.

Q: *And cardiac muscle?*
A: Cardiac muscle, also involuntary, is found within the heart. It is a kind of cross between smooth and skeletal muscle. Cardiac muscle is responsible for keeping your heart beating and pumping blood throughout the body without your having to do anything about it.

Q: *How do these muscles actually work?*
A: There are over six hundred voluntary skeletal muscles in the body. One example is the biceps in the front of the upper arm. When muscles like these contract, they shorten and produce movement by pulling on the bones.

The biceps muscle is attached to the shoulder and elbow, so when it contracts and pulls the bones together, the arm flexes. The forearm is brought closer to the upper arm. Then, to straighten the arm out, the opposing muscle group, the triceps muscle, contracts as the biceps relaxes and lengthens. Then we have the opposite movement, extension, as the humerus or upper arm bone and the radius and ulna, the forearm bones, are moved further apart.

Within the intestinal tract, smooth muscle contraction moves food along. Smooth muscle contraction changes the pressure within the blood vessels. There are quite a few different types of smooth muscle in the body that produce different actions.

Q: *How does the body make energy and create movement?*
A: The body makes energy by converting food into the chemical energy currency of the body, which is called ATP (adenosine triphosphate). An elaborate series of reactions converts the food we eat into ATP. Within the cells, food can be burned for energy with or without oxygen in order to produce ATP.

When food is broken down into energy without oxygen, the process is called anaerobic metabolism, with anaerobic meaning without oxygen. This action produces a small number of ATP molecules as the chemical bonds of our food are broken down.

Then food can be further broken down in the mitochondria of cells, which are sub-units of cells specifically for energy production. Food components from protein, carbohydrates, and fat can all be transported into the mitochondria and burned in the presence of oxygen to produce energy in the form of ATP. This process involving oxygen is called aerobic metabolism, and results in a much greater production of ATP—95 percent of the body's energy.

So basically, the body uses chemical reactions to release energy from the chemical bonds from the foods we eat, creating ATP.

Q: *What happens when you want to be physically active?*
A: When you want to use your muscles to perform an activity, your body breaks down ATP and converts it into ADP (adenosine diphosphate), which releases energy. Creatine phosphate donates its phosphate group to ADP to regenerate the ATP and provide further fuel for energy and activity. ADP combines with creatine phosphate to form ATP and creatine. During recovery from intense activity, ATP levels increase and ATP can donate a phosphate group to creatine to regenerate creatine phosphate.

Q: *What do our muscles need in order to stay healthy?*
A: To generate energy and repair worn out and damaged tissue,

Lisa: Creatine for Feminine Curves

When Lisa, a 36-year-old graphic designer, first came to me, she was interested in losing weight. First we reviewed her health history and then took some measurements. Using bioelectric impedance analysis to assess Lisa's body composition, I found that she had an elevated body fat percentage and abnormally low muscle mass.

I explained the results of the analysis to Lisa and asked what her goal was. She replied, "To lose fifteen pounds." I said, "No, it isn't. Your real goal is to look better and to feel healthier."

"What's the difference?" she asked me. I told her that body composition was very important and not only would she benefit from losing fat, but she would also benefit from building muscle.

I designed a program for Lisa that would help her shed fat and build lean shapely muscle. It consisted of a balanced whole-food diet, weight training, aerobic exercise, weight loss supplements, and creatine.

After staying on this program for six weeks, Lisa returned to my office looking far better. She had more curves and a smaller waistline. Although she had only lost four pounds, she told me that her friends kept telling her how good she looked.

We repeated the body composition analysis and found that Lisa had actually lost eight pounds of fat and put on four pounds of muscle.

Lisa's starting body composition is typical of many overweight women and is called "sarcopenic obesity," which means both too little muscle and too much fat. It is an unhealthy combination which makes a person appear even heavier than they really are.

So weight loss is not the true goal for such people. Instead, it is the type of weight you lose that is significant. Contrary to popular opinion, just going on a diet and losing weight does not guarantee you will achieve your real goal of a more attractive appearance.

The best way to approach this condition is to combine weight training and creatine with a sensible diet. By doing that, you will be much more likely to lose fat and build muscle mass. Remember that it is healthy muscles that give women a lean, curvy appearance.

So if you want to burn more calories efficiently, you may want to think about putting on some muscle. And as Lisa's experience shows, nothing builds muscle as safely as a combination of weight training and creatine.

muscles need good nutrition and oxygen. You also need good circulation in order to deliver oxygen and nutrients to the muscles. In other words, the blood vessels have to be healthy and able to deliver blood with oxygen and nutrients. Muscle cells also need to have their metabolic waste removed by the circulatory system in order to stay healthy. And like all tissue in the body, muscle cells also need to be stimulated by a healthy mix of hormones and other cellular messaging chemicals.

You also need exercise—the muscles have to be used. If the muscles are not challenged, they will atrophy, or become smaller and weaker. So muscles need regular exercise, specifically progressive resistance exercise. That refers to increasing the intensity of exercise over time, which is important because the muscles will adapt to whatever stress they undergo, so the next time they experience the same work load, they can deal with it more easily.

Q: So the work load needs to be increased?
A: Yes. If the work load is kept the same, the muscles won't grow and become stronger and more efficient. They need to be challenged with progressively greater work loads.

Q: What about rest?
A: That's very important. Muscles definitely need some rest.

They need to be exercised, but they also need a chance to recover from activity and repair themselves.

Q: *What do muscles need for growth?*
A: Muscles need adequate rest, time to recover, good nutrition, and adequate protein. And they also need stress. In other words, they need to be worked hard with exercise. Specifically, they require high-intensity resistance exercise and that is accomplished most commonly by weight training.

Q: *How does weight training work?*
A: Muscles have to work against heavy resistance so that they are stressed over a short period of time in order to cause micro-tears within their fibers. The body repairs these small tears and compensates for them by increasing protein synthesis and making the muscle fibers even bigger.

Q: *What type of exercise does this?*
A: Endurance exercise cannot accomplish this. It has to be anaerobic, high-resistance exercise like weight training, where people are doing about ten repetitions to failure, working the muscle until they can't accomplish another repetition.

Q: *But they can't do that every day?*
A: No, they can't. The muscles need rest. Individuals vary as to how much rest they need. Some people can train a few times a week or even more frequently, and I have known others who had to wait as long as ten days between workouts for enough recovery time after an all-out workout.

Q: *How does each person know how long to rest?*
A: Each individual has to determine it by trial and error. You have to be aware of how you respond, how your strength is dur-

ing the workout. You can also consult a knowledgeable health care professional and have lab tests that can help determine if you are over training. In addition, there are symptoms of over-training you have to watch for.

Q: What are some of the signs that you are over-training?
A: There are quite a few, including mood changes, feeling sick, waking up with a rapid heartbeat, and of course, seeing your performance deteriorate while you are exercising.

You can also take a lab test of immune system function using a saliva specimen and if you are over-training, your immune system will be depressed. Analysis of stress hormone levels, again through saliva specimens, is another gauge of over-training.

Q: What about the muscles' need for protein?
A: It's very important. Some vegetarian diets may not supply optimum quantities of complete protein. And with aging, the body has an increased need for protein. So the body must get enough protein in order to maintain the muscles—that's what muscles are made of. We need enough protein both to repair the damaged muscle fibers that result from physical activity, and to help the muscles grow.

Q: What about the influence of genetics on muscular strength and athletic performance?
A: Genetics is an important factor. We all have a certain potential within our genetic makeup and what we do consciously or unconsciously when we take part in competitive athletics is to try to optimize our genetic expression. The way we do that is through training. We stress the muscles with heavy loads over a short period of time and try to make the most of whatever capabilities we have inherited.

Q: *What else influences athletic performance?*
A: As we have said, adequate rest, good nutrition, healthy levels of essential hormones and the level of creatine phosphate in the muscle cells. If there's a greater level of creatine phosphate, then there's a greater potential for energy production, which translates into increased muscle contraction and strength.

Q: *What happens when the muscles are injured?*
A: There are different ways that muscles can become injured. With a common injury called a strain, there is actually tearing of the tissue. With a severe strain, the tearing of the muscle and connective tissue can even tear the muscle completely through—that's called a rupture. That type of injury requires surgery.

Sometimes even tears that are less than a rupture also require surgery. The mildest of tears heal with new muscle cells, but most muscle strains involve the deposition of scar tissue into the injured muscle, so the muscle does not return to its pre-injury state. It has scar tissue in place of some of the muscle fibers and scar tissue is not as strong or flexible and doesn't have the contractile ability of muscle cells. So one goal of injury rehabilitation is to make the healing scar tissue as strong and as flexible as possible.

Q: *How do you know when you have a serious injury?*
A: Serious injuries are usually associated with pain, redness, swelling, heat, and disability. With a bad injury, you won't be able to move the part of the body that is injured, and over time, it can lead to atrophy of the muscle. For example, if a limb is immobilized in a cast, brace or sling for a period of time, you will get muscle atrophy, and you can get it pretty quickly. This can also happen with the chronically ill or disabled elderly who are forced to spend a lot of time immobilized in bed. And as you will see later on,

research shows that supplementation with creatine can reduce muscle atrophy that occurs with this type of lack of movement.

Q: If you take creatine in supplemental form, does your body stop making its own creatine?
A: If you ingest more creatine than your body needs, your body will stop making its own supplies. Once creatine supplementation is stopped, the body begins making it again.

Q: How does creatine affect the muscles in terms of strength and growth?
A: Creatine leads to regeneration of ATP within muscle cells and ATP levels determine the cells' ability to contract. In this way, when creatine increases ATP levels, it leads to increased muscular contraction, increased muscular strength, increased ability to handle work loads, and increased ability to exercise longer and recover more quickly after a bout of exercise.

Creatine phosphate levels increase ATP and that leads to greater and longer maximal physical efforts. So the bottom line is: creatine increases strength.

As for muscles, creatine works in a couple of different ways in the muscles cells. It increases the water content of the muscle cell and that in itself is probably responsible for some increase in muscle size. Creatine also apparently increases protein synthesis and may reduce protein breakdown within muscle cells. The end result is that muscles get bigger.

Points to Remember

- The body has three different types of muscle: skeletal, smooth, and cardiac.
- Skeletal muscle is connected to bones and is responsible for voluntary movements, which you consciously control.

- The body makes energy by converting food into ATP, the fuel for cells. In turn, ATP is converted into ADP, releasing energy.
- Healthy muscles need good nutrition, oxygen, rest, and challenging activity.
- High-intensity resistance exercise, most often performed in the activity of weight training, is essential for muscle growth.
- People vary in their physical needs for exercise and recovery time. Sometimes a health care professional and lab tests can help to determine your individual needs.
- Genetic factors can also have an influence on individual response to physical activity.
- There are varying degrees of muscle injuries, the more serious requiring surgery.
- Mild muscle tears heal with scar tissue, but the muscles do not automatically return to their pre-injury strength.
- Muscle injuries leading to even short-term immobilization can cause muscles to atrophy. Supplemental creatine can minimize this atrophy.
- Creatine helps to increase protein synthesis and foster muscle growth and strength.

CHAPTER FOUR

How Did Creatine Become So Popular?

IN THIS CHAPTER, you will learn about the history of creatine: when it was discovered and how it has been used in the past; how creatine was secretly used by Eastern Bloc countries to enhance athletic performance; how widely creatine is used in professional and amateur sports today; and whether you or all the others using creatine supplements can feel certain that it is safe and effective.

Q: How was creatine originally discovered?
A: In 1832, a French organic chemist named Michel-Eugéne Chevreul discovered creatine by extracting it from meat. In fact, the name creatine, which he gave his new discovery, comes from the Greek word for flesh. Some time after that, scientists found that there was more creatine in the muscles of foxes killed in the wild than in domestic foxes, and they concluded that the greater amount of physical activity among wild foxes lead to more creatine in their bodies.

Q: When was synthetic creatine first developed?
A: In the 1950s, scientists learned to synthesize creatine in the lab, and that is the form of creatine we now have in supplements.

Q: What were the first uses for creatine supplements?
A: In the beginning, creatine was used for medical conditions. For example, it was used for a genetic metabolic disorder called gyrate atrophy, which affects the eye and type II muscle fibers. This condition involves excess buildup of the amino acid, ornithine, which inhibits creatine synthesis in the body. So people with gyrate atrophy have lower creatine phosphate levels in their muscle cells, and their muscles can shrink and become very weak. As demonstrated by a study reported in *The New England Journal of Medicine* in 1981, giving creatine supplements to people with this condition causes muscle fibers to grow larger and also become considerably strengthened. (See Chapter Five for further discussion on creatine's health benefits.)

Q: When was creatine first used as a sports supplement?
A: In the late 1960s and early 1970s, scientists began to discover that, under certain conditions, creatine could enhance athletic performance. There are reports that beginning in the late 1960s, creatine was secretly given to athletes in the Eastern Bloc countries by government-sponsored agencies, in combination with highly dangerous anabolic steroids (see Chapter Ten), to make these athletes more competitive.

After the use of these muscle-enhancers became widespread, suspicions were aroused in Olympic competitions, most notably with the East German women swimmers, since competitors and officials from other countries observed a sudden and dramatic increase in the athletes' size and muscular strength. Since that time, anabolic steroids have been implicated and banned in many sports, including Olympic competition.

Q: *Has the use of creatine also been restricted?*
A: Creatine is not banned by any amateur or professional sports organization and no scientific study has ever found creatine to have any dangerous side effects like steroids.

Q: *So creatine is widely used in sports today?*
A: Yes, that's right. Its use is especially widespread in sports like football, baseball, and weight lifting, where short bursts of intense energy are often needed and where creatine would therefore be effective.

Q: *Is creatine also widely used by amateur athletes who are interested in better sports or exercise performance?*
A: Definitely. There are studies that show this to be true. For example, one study of collegiate athletes found that overall, 28 percent had used creatine—48 percent of the men and 4 percent of the women studied. In surveys of high school athletes, results indicate that as many as half of all senior football players have tried creatine and more than 16 percent of high school athletes have used it.

Q: *How do people hear about creatine?*
A: In the study of collegiate athletes, most of them had heard about creatine through their friends and had first tried it in high school. Of course, there is also a lot of advertising for different creatine products in magazines, newspapers, and on the internet, and you can see many of these products when you shop in health food stores and some supermarkets.

Q: *How did you first hear about creatine?*
A: I think it was in a book I read in the early 1990s about ergogenic (tending to increase work output) aids. At that time, there weren't a lot of studies on creatine, but there was one study

showing that creatine supplementation increased the creatine content of muscles. I found that of great interest.

Q: *Did you use it right away?*
A: No. By the time I decided to try it, I had known about it for a while, had seen quite a few studies indicating that it was both safe and effective, and had also seen a lot of advertisements from supplement companies and articles in muscle magazines.

Q: *To date, have you seen any scientific evidence of any kind of danger in using creatine?*
A: No. There have been anecdotal reports with people saying they took creatine and then had problems such as kidney damage or heat stroke, but no link has ever been proven between creatine use and any serious side effects or long-term health problems (see Chapter Nine). So until somebody completes a study that proves a direct cause-and-effect, as far as I know creatine is very safe.

Q: *Then you feel completely confident about creatine's safety?*
A: Absolutely, as long as the creatine product is a quality supplement, free of impurities. The safety of creatine has been more extensively studied than any other performance-enhancing nutritional supplement. I think that if you cut away the media hype, the rumors, and the lack of hard information, you will find that creatine is extremely safe and has a very low incidence of minor side effects.

Points to Remember

• Creatine was discovered in 1832 and has been used as a nutritional supplement since the 1960s.

- Creatine is used to treat a variety of medical disorders.
- Creatine was used in combination with anabolic steroids in Eastern Bloc countries in the 1960s and 1970s.
- Anabolic steroids are dangerous and have been widely banned; creatine is considered safe and has never been banned.
- Creatine is widely used by amateur and professional athletes, especially in the specific sports where it is most effective.
- The major way people hear about creatine is word-of-mouth from friends who have tried it.
- No scientific studies have proven any links between creatine and any serious side effects or diseases.
- Hundreds of studies indicate that creatine is a very safe and effective supplement.

CHAPTER FIVE

The Health Benefits of Creatine

CREATINE IS MUCH more than a muscle-enhancing supplement. Before you learn how it can help with your athletic performance, you should know something about its effectiveness with certain medical conditions, as well as the ongoing studies that may discover additional medical applications in the future.

Q: Is it true that creatine is used to help treat different medical problems?
A: Yes, creatine supplementation has been found to benefit people suffering from neuromuscular afflictions, heart disease, and other medical conditions. Taking creatine can also be considered a preventive measure, since it has a role in helping to keep people healthy and functional as they grow older.

Q: Why does creatine have beneficial effects on these medical conditions?
A: To appreciate the true importance of creatine to overall health, you have to understand the central role of energy pro-

duction in normal metabolism. When one thinks of creatine's effect in the body, muscle contraction usually comes to mind. In reality, virtually every biochemical reaction and physiologic process in the body requires energy. Creatine plays an important role in the production of energy. All cellular functions require energy and nothing works as well as it should without a sufficient source of energy. Lower creatine phosphate levels in cells cause sub-optimal metabolism and health.

Q: *What happens in the body when there is insufficient energy production?*
A: One of the many consequences of sub-optimal cellular energy is weakening of the cells. Cells are more likely to be damaged or die. For example, when a cell's blood supply is interrupted, oxygen delivery is impaired and aerobic energy production within the cell drops, causing cell damage. If creatine phosphate levels are high within the cell, ATP levels can be maintained longer, protecting the cell until oxygen is circulated to it again.

Such a scenario of interrupted blood supply and impaired oxidative metabolism is not uncommon, particularly in the elderly. When it affects the brain, it is called a "transient ischemic attack." If brain cells sustain damage, that is called a "stroke." Based on animal research, it appears that creatine supplementation may offer protection against these events.

Q: *How does creatine protect the brain?*
A: Protection against damage from traumatic brain injury is another valuable potential application for creatine supplementation. Millions of people suffer brain injuries every year in sports, recreational activities, and in traffic and other accidents. Repeated concussions in sports such as soccer and football are very common and may also result in brain injuries. Again, by helping maintain cellular energy production and by stabilizing

cell membranes, supplemental creatine can reduce damage from such injuries. So athletes may also be protecting their brains when they use creatine to build more muscle.

Q: Are there any studies dealing with creatine's effects on these types of injuries?
A: Yes. A 2002 animal study that appeared in the journal *Spinal Cord* was designed to evaluate the influence of creatine supplementation on spinal cord injury. The study found that after experimental spinal cord contusions, creatine-supplemented animals experienced less structural damage and retained better function than non-supplemented animals. The authors of the study concluded, "Our results favor a pretreatment of patients with creatine for neuroprotection in cases of elective intramedullary spinal surgery. Further studies are needed to evaluate the benefit of immediate creatine administration in case of acute spinal cord or brain injury."

Q: How can creatine's effects on muscle benefit the elderly?
A: Studies have shown that creatine increases muscle mass and strength in the elderly, especially when supplements are combined with regular physical activity. Having more strength can mean the difference between being bedridden or wheelchair-bound and being ambulatory and able to move around freely on your own. Greater strength is critical in emergency situations, like trying to avoid a fall. Studies on weight training have proven that even people in their nineties can benefit, so combining exercise with creatine can produce great results in older men and women.

Q: Would you advocate weight training equipment for nursing homes?
A: Yes, of course. One of the most important things people can

do for their health is to weight train. With aging, there's a tendency to lose muscle mass and become weaker. In fact, a Tufts University study found that the number-one factor correlating with aging is the loss of muscle mass.

So the importance of restoring strength and muscle in the elderly can't be overemphasized. I would really like to see older people and those in nursing homes undergoing weight training and using creatine supplements under their doctors' supervision. I believe the results would be beneficial and might really surprise everyone.

Q: *Is it true that creatine can also benefit people who are recovering from immobilization due to injury or surgery?*
A: Yes, that's right. One 2001 study involved leg casts placed on healthy people for two weeks. Half the subjects were given creatine and the other half were given a placebo (a look-alike substitute with no active ingredient). They found that during the rehabilitation period after the casts were removed, the size and power of the quadriceps muscle recovered much more quickly in the creatine group.

Q: *What do we know about high cholesterol and triglyceride levels in the body and their dangers?*
A: We know there is a relationship between elevated total cholesterol levels in the blood and the risk of cardiovascular disease. There is also an association between levels of HDL (good cholesterol) and levels of LDL (bad cholesterol.) The higher the HDL, the better off you are; the higher the LDL, the greater your risk of cardiovascular disease. VLDL cholesterol is another form that is unhealthy in high concentrations.

The same is true for triglycerides (dangerous blood fats that can clog arteries). As with LDL cholesterol, higher triglycerides are associated with an increased risk of cardiovascular disease.

Brian: Gaining a Muscular Edge

While preparing for an East Coast bodybuilding competition several years ago, Brian consulted me for nutritional advice. A 27-year-old fireman, Brian was in great shape and had trained very hard.

Brian explained that he was worried that his attempt to shed as much body fat as possible was also going to cause excessive muscle loss. I suggested that Brian try creatine to see if the supplement would help him to preserve and build muscle, while helping him lose body fat.

After the loading phase, Brian reported that he immediately felt an increase in energy, which had been lagging before. He noticed that his muscles began to rapidly fill out and become more vascular.

Brian was especially happy when he went on to win the competition, taking first place in his class. Brian continued to use creatine for future competitions, with many additional successes.

Q: What have studies shown about the effects of creatine on cholesterol and triglyceride levels?
A: A 1996 study found that after eight weeks of creatine supplementation, the subjects had an average 5 to 6 percent reduction in total cholesterol and a 22 to 23 percent reduction in triglycerides and VLDL cholesterol. And four weeks after the creatine was stopped, there was still a reduction in triglyceride levels, although the cholesterol returned to its previous levels.

Q: Have there been similar studies that included exercise?
A: Yes. One study found that resistance training, with or without creatine, did not affect lipid (cholesterol and triglyceride) levels. This study used a lower (5 grams) maintenance dose than studies that found a beneficial effect on blood lipids (which used 10 grams per day).

Another study in 2001 looked at subjects who either took creatine and did not exercise, took creatine and did weight training, or took a placebo and did weight training. They found that after twenty-eight days, the group that took creatine and did not exercise, and the group that took a placebo and did exercise both showed no change in cholesterol levels. But the group that took creatine and exercised had close to a 10 percent reduction in total cholesterol.

We should point out that it is not desirable for everyone to have a reduction in cholesterol levels. Cholesterol, despite its bad reputation, is essential for good health. Vitamin D, bile acids, cell membranes, and steroid hormones are all made from cholesterol. I believe that creatine will help to lower lipids for people whose levels are too high, but will not lower them for those who already have desirable levels.

Q: *Can we conclude that exercise and creatine together are the key?*
A: Yes. While there are some benefits to using creatine alone, the full benefits appear to involve a regular combination of creatine and exercise.

Q: *Creatine has been used for people with certain serious medical disorders. Can you discuss some of them, such as Lou Gehrig's disease?*
A: Lou Gehrig's disease, also known as amyotrophic lateral sclerosis, involves muscle atrophy due to degeneration of the spinal cord. In one study, creatine provided a temporary benefit to patients with this disease, increasing their strength and resistance to fatigue. But after six months, these benefits seemed to wear off, so I think more studies need to be done. Future studies might find some benefit by cycling creatine on and off.

Q: What about other neuromuscular diseases such as Parkinson's disease, muscular dystrophy, mitochondrial cytopathy, and Huntington's disease? Is there any evidence that creatine supplements can help?

A: Yes, creatine has been studied with some of these conditions and found to be helpful. For example, one 2000 study of muscular dystrophy patients found a mild but significant improvement in muscle strength and daily life activities after eight weeks of creatine supplementation.

Another study in 1999 concluded that "short-term creatine monohydrate increased high intensity strength significantly in patients with neuromuscular disease." Myasthenia gravis, an autoimmune neuromuscular disease, and McArdle's disease, an inherited glycogen metabolism disorder, are two other conditions associated with lower creatine levels in the body. Both these disorders can apparently be helped by creatine supplementation.

Studies on animals with a disorder similar to Parkinson's in humans showed much less brain dopamine loss and cell death when the test subjects were given creatine. Dopamine is the neurotransmitter that people with Parkinson's disease have in insufficient levels. So based on animal studies, creatine may give some protection against the development of Parkinson's.

Q: Can creatine help with Alzheimer's disease?

A: It is very possible. When brain cells don't produce enough energy, they become weaker and more vulnerable to toxic insult, and therefore more likely to die. So it's very important that brain cells have constant production of adequate energy levels. Based on animal studies, creatine may help to accomplish this.

Creatine has been found to protect brain cells against certain neurotoxins and to protect the hippocampal neurons, which are in the area of the brain that is most affected by Alzheimer's.

In these animal studies of Parkinson's and Alzheimer's, the animals that were given creatine supplements had higher intracellular creatine and creatine phosphate levels than non-supplemented animals, which could play a role in protection against brain injury from toxins. Of course, we need much more documentation and studies with humans to prove a direct cause and effect, but the apparently protective role of creatine in these disorders is definitely a hopeful sign.

Finally, animal models of Huntington's disease (another degenerative brain condition) have also found creatine supplementation to provide significant benefits.

Q: Can creatine supplements help with inherited diseases, including those that result in the body being unable to make creatine?
A: Studies have shown that people with inherited defects in creatine synthesis have decreased levels of creatine and creatine phosphate in muscle and brain cells, resulting in impaired physical and mental development. By taking supplemental creatine, people with these conditions can raise their cellular creatine levels and develop more normally, both physically and mentally.

Q: How can creatine be helpful for people with heart disease?
A: Studies have demonstrated that intravenous use of creatine phosphate can reduce ventricular fibrillation in patients with ischemic heart disease. In regard to oral creatine (the most common form of supplements), its use has been evaluated in patients with congestive heart failure and these patients have benefited with better exercise performance, both in strength and endurance.

An additional study found that people with diseased hearts—dilated cardiomyopathy, or enlarged hearts that don't work properly—had 50 percent less total creatine when compared with healthy hearts, and 30 percent fewer creatine transporters, the proteins that transport creatine into the cells.

Q: Can you explain the connection between creatine and homocysteine?
A: That is an area of current interest to creatine researchers. Homocysteine is a toxic amino acid that we all have within our bodies. When levels of homocysteine climb above a certain point, it becomes dangerous. Elevated homocysteine has been associated with about fifty degenerative diseases including cardiovascular disease, some cancers, Alzheimer's disease, Parkinson's disease, and memory impairment. So far, studies on the effect of creatine on homocysteine levels have been mixed, with one animal study showing a significant benefit from creatine and one human study showing no benefit. So we will have to wait and see what future studies may reveal.

Q: Are there any other medical uses for creatine?
A: A common complaint of renal failure patients undergoing hemodialysis is muscle cramping. Research published in November 2002 found that supplemental creatine reduced muscle cramping 60 percent more than placebo treatment.

Another likely role for creatine is indicated by the results of a recently published animal study. Corticosteroids are medications commonly prescribed to patients for reducing inflammation that accompanies injuries and conditions including autoimmune diseases like arthritis and allergies. Two of the adverse side effects of corticosteroids are impairment of growth and loss of muscle mass.

Supplemental creatine was investigated to see if it could have a beneficial effect on these unwanted side effects of corticosteroids. The study found that the animals given only corticosteroids experienced less weight gain and the animals given creatine along with the corticosteroids had more normal growth and developed larger type II muscle fibers. It is quite possible that these results can also be obtained in human studies, but we will have to wait to confirm that.

The results of this study may have even greater significance. Individuals suffering from chronic mental-emotional, physical or physiologic stress develop elevated levels of the stress hormone cortisol. Cortisol is the body's natural corticosteroid. It follows then, that creatine supplementation may reduce some of the adverse physiological effects of chronic stress.

Q: *Does creatine affect carbohydrate metabolism?*
A: That is another area that needs more investigation. But there is some evidence indicating that creatine may have a beneficial impact on the way the body metabolizes carbohydrates. That can be very important for certain health conditions, like diabetes, as well as many age-related diseases and even the aging process itself. This finding may also apply to the one out of three Americans who has the condition called insulin resistance, which impairs metabolism and results in poor health and obesity.

Q: *Will taking creatine supplements improve the health of the average person?*
A: There have been many studies on the benefits of creatine and many more remain to be done. But we can conclude that creatine has many benefits that extend beyond sports performance. Some of these studies are conflicting and not every study finds that creatine shows benefits. You also have to take into consideration that every individual is biochemically unique and what works for one person may not work for another.

But looking at these studies overall, it is apparent that creatine has many potential benefits, even for those who do not combine the supplement with physical exercise or participation in sports.

So it is my opinion that not only people in sports and people with some of the specific health conditions we have mentioned, but average people may very well feel better and also protect themselves against declining health as they age by taking creatine. And the main reason can be found in the potential for creatine to preserve muscle and strength as people grow older. That is one of its most important benefits.

Q: So even a couch potato could benefit?
A: It's certainly possible. But it is important to remember that the very best results come from a combination of creatine supplementation and weight training.

Points to Remember

- Creatine can be helpful for treating many medical disorders, including Lou Gehrig's disease, muscular dystrophy, myasthenia gravis, McArdle's disease, gyrate atrophy, mitochondrial cytopathy, and possibly Parkinson's, Huntington's and Alzheimer's diseases, and cardiovascular disease.
- Creatine increases muscle mass and strength in the elderly, especially in combination with regular exercise.
- Creatine can help patients recover after surgery and casting by rebuilding weakened muscles.
- Creatine has been found to lower total cholesterol.
- Creatine also lowers triglycerides, which are associated with cardiovascular disease.
- Creatine supplements can help people with certain genetic disorders to maintain normal creatine phosphate levels.
- Creatine supplements may benefit everyone, even if they don't exercise.
- Creatine in combination with regular exercise, especially weight training, yields the best results.

CHAPTER SIX

How Does Creatine Enhance Sports Performance?

NOT EVERY TYPE of sport or physical activity benefits from creatine. So before you buy creatine and begin using it, you need to know if taking creatine could result in better performance in your specific sport or physical activity. In this chapter, we will talk about which individual sports benefit and do not benefit from creatine supplements and why; how the effects of creatine can differ in men and women; and how official sports organizations view creatine.

Q: What is the difference between aerobic and anaerobic exercise and which type or types can benefit from creatine supplementation?
A: Aerobic exercise refers to exercise that requires oxygen. Anaerobic exercise refers to exercise that does not require oxygen. Creatine is primarily helpful with the anaerobic type of exercise.

Aerobic exercise is extended or long-term activity and involves steady, low-intensity energy, such as the kind we find in long-distance running and bicycling, as well as jogging and walking.

Anaerobic exercise is short-term activity and involves short bursts of very high-intensity energy, such as the kind we find in weight lifting, wrestling, football, and sprinting.

But not all forms of exercise or sports are either one kind or the other. There are times when aerobic and anaerobic activities are mixed. For example, in basketball you may need a short-term burst of anaerobic energy to jump to dunk a basket, but you also need long-term steady aerobic energy to run around the court for most of the game.

Q: How are creatine stores in the body involved in producing energy?
A: Anaerobic exercise, which is most often helped by creatine, proceeds with the generation of energy produced without oxygen by ATP and from ATP regeneration from creatine phosphate. These sources of energy last for up to thirty seconds. Creatine phosphate is mostly involved for the first five to ten seconds with a lesser effect up to thirty seconds.

After the creatine sources are depleted, the next energy system that is used with high-intensity exercise is anaerobic glycolysis, the burning of sugars without oxygen. That system is good for up to seven minutes.

For longer activities of lesser intensity, there is also oxidative phosphorylation or aerobic metabolism, that involves burning carbohydrates, fats, and amino acids with oxygen.

There is an overlap among these different systems, but initially, with very high-intensity exercise, ATP and creatine phosphate are what the body uses for driving these activities.

Q: Then anaerobic exercise is the type that really benefits from creatine supplements?
A: Yes. It's with anaerobic activities that creatine phosphate is directly involved. When you supplement with creatine, you

increase your cells' creatine levels and a good proportion of that creatine becomes creatine phosphate, which is the active molecule involved in energy production.

There is also some evidence that creatine supplementation can help with exercise that goes beyond the five to ten second range. Exercise lasting from 30 to 150 seconds and even exercise up to and beyond three minutes may also benefit from higher cellular levels of creatine phosphate.

Q: How does creatine also help with this longer term exercise?
A: It appears that creatine supplementation has beneficial effects on how the body uses its other energy systems. There are several studies that suggest that creatine supplementation delays anaerobic glycolysis. Creatine supplementation also leads to a significant increase in glycogen storage, which translates into more fuel for prolonged exercise. Additionally, higher cellular creatine phosphate levels may improve buffering of the acidity that is a byproduct of anaerobic glycolysis. Thus, more lactic acid could accumulate before resulting in muscular exhaustion. Creatine also appears to help the body utilize oxygen more efficiently for production of longer, sustained energy levels.

Q: Which specific sports benefit the most from creatine supplements?
A: Athletes in many different sports may benefit from creatine, especially when training or competing in the sports that require maximal or near-maximal exertion over short periods of time and also include repetitive bursts of energy. Activities of this type include weight lifting, power lifting, bodybuilding, football, wrestling, boxing, hockey, tennis, volleyball, squash, team handball, basketball, skiing, soccer, lacrosse, rugby, arm wrestling, short-distance bicycling, rowing, baseball, short-distance swimming, and track and field events.

Tim: Better Health—What's It Worth?

Tim, a 55-year-old tennis instructor, consulted me for an evaluation and treatment of a variety of symptoms, including extreme weakness, heart palpitations, heat intolerance, headaches, and tingling in his hands. Tim told me that he had always been underweight, and when he came in, he weighed only 129-1/2 pounds, despite his height of 5'11".

After taking his health history, I evaluated Tim using various laboratory tests and based on the results, suggested stress reduction, a change of diet, and the addition of nutritional supplements.

Tim followed the program I outlined for him and after a few months, we saw a gradual improvement, but the weakness and fatigue persisted. I then recommended that Tim add creatine monohydrate to his program. Tim was surprised and told me that a friend, who was a former Junior World Weight Lifting champion, had also recommended creatine to him.

Tim used 5 grams of creatine with a cup of water once a day. After only a day or two, he reported feeling increased energy and a quicker gait. But Tim also experienced increased hunger and thirst, which he attributed to the addition of creatine in his diet. After a few weeks, Tim decided to stop using creatine because, as he said, "I don't want to spend any extra time or money on food and water."

Since giving up creatine, Tim has noticed that his energy is not the same, and he is now thinking again about possibly going back to creatine supplements.

Q: Does creatine also help with activities of longer duration?
A: Yes. Some studies have found creatine to benefit high-intensity activities up to and beyond three minutes in duration.

I think the contribution of creatine supplementation to enhancing performance in activities of longer duration are well-illustrated by the results of kayak ergometer tests as reported in the *European Journal of Applied Physiology* in 1998. Compared to the elite kayakers taking a placebo, those supplementing with creatine had increases in work capacity of 16.2 percent at 90 seconds, 13.6 percent at 150 seconds and 6.6 percent at 300 seconds. So we can see that activities of longer duration benefited from creatine supplementation but to a lesser degree.

The conclusion is that creatine benefits can also apply to endurance sports where short bursts of energy are involved. So, for example, if you are going all out in the last few seconds of a long-distance race, you may be helped by extra stores of creatine and for some people, that can even be the difference between a silver and gold medal.

Q: *What specific movements in these sports are helped most by creatine?*
A: The primary movements where creatine has been proven helpful are lifting, sprinting, and rowing. Theoretically, creatine should also help with throwing, hitting, and kicking.

Q: *What are some of the sports where creatine is either not helpful or only minimally helpful?*
A: As we have pointed out, creatine is not very beneficial in long-term endurance sports, such as marathon running or long-distance swimming or bicycling. Creatine could also be a detriment because it usually causes an increase in weight. The same is true of athletes in sports involving jumping, such as some track and field events. The increased weight may make it more difficult for an athlete to perform the activity, so this negative aspect of creatine may outweigh its benefits in that particular sport. For instance, weight gain could be a potentially serious drawback for swimmers or athletes involved in jumping.

Several studies have found creatine to benefit jumping performance, but other studies have not. Some individuals in these sports will have an overall performance benefit from creatine and others will not. Therefore, it is best to experiment with creatine during the off season to find out whether it works to your benefit.

Q: Does everyone gain weight when they use creatine?
A: Apparently no, not everyone does. So we can't say that creatine is either totally good or bad for aerobic sports. But we do know that creatine is not going to be as helpful for the long-distance endurance sports that require lower-intensity efforts for longer periods of time, because of the increase in body weight and because creatine's major effect is helping with short bursts of intense energy rather than with long-term steady energy.

Q: You are a former competitive weight lifter. What do you know about the effects of creatine on this sport?
A: There is a lot of data from many studies on the impact of creatine supplements on lifting weights. And it appears that creatine is very beneficial for power lifters and weight lifters. Most of these studies have found benefits in maximal strength, that is, the ability to lift a heavy weight one time. Many studies have also shown that creatine boosts the ability to lift a near-maximal weight several times, which has tremendous application to improving training intensity. The end result is increased strength and ultimately performance, in any sport with a strength component.

Q: Can you provide some details about one of these studies?
A: Yes. Researchers who authored a 2002 study, which was published in *Medicine and Science in Sports and Exercise,* found that after five days of creatine supplementation, the placebo group had no increase in their one-repetition maximum weight half squat, but the group that got creatine had an 11 percent increase. Other activities where we have evidence that creatine can be helpful are cycling sprints, running sprints, swimming

sprints, skating sprints and jumping. Several studies, including a 1999 study published in the *Journal of Sports Medicine and Physical Fitness*, have demonstrated increased sprinting performance with the use of creatine supplements.

It should be noted that not all studies have found creatine supplementation to benefit sprinting and jumping. Perhaps the increase in body weight that results from using creatine is the explanation.

Q: What about bodybuilders, the group of athletes that first popularized the muscle-boosting benefits of creatine?
A: Because of their need for increased muscle mass, bodybuilders can really benefit from creatine. Many studies show an increase in body weight, with the increase in the form of desirable fat-free mass. Studies have also shown increases in intracellular water content in muscle cells, as well as in size of the muscle cells, both of which are helpful for bodybuilders.

In other words, bodybuilders get bigger and more defined when they use creatine. A 2000 study which appeared in *Medicine and Science in Sports and Exercise* found that after six weeks of resistance training, there was no change in the placebo group, but the group taking creatine had a measurable increase in the size of the upper arm.

Q: When creatine causes weight gain, isn't it because of water retention?
A: Initially, the weight gain produced by creatine is apparently due to muscle cells taking up more water. I view this as a positive change, since biological aging and failing health are associated with just the opposite change—a decrease in intracellular water.

Creatine's impact on body weight, however, is not limited to water retention. There are several different lines of evidence indicating that creatine increases protein synthesis and actual growth of the muscle cells. Creatine may also reduce protein breakdown. Additionally, the increased strength and stamina that result from creatine supplementation allow you to train harder and thereby, over time, to build more muscle.

Q: Baseball is one of the sports where creatine is widely used. What role does creatine play with baseball players?
A: One study involving creatine and the velocity of pitchers' fast balls found that creatine had no effect. But that was just one study and other studies may have different results.

In baseball, it seems that creatine might possibly be helpful for relief pitchers, for runners sprinting, or for an outfielder making a quick throw to get the ball to the infield. All of these movements are quick bursts of intense energy and increased creatine stores should be helpful for such movements.

Q: Exactly what does creatine do to help athletes in the sports where it is effective?
A: As we have seen, creatine supplements increase muscle creatine phosphate levels, allowing for increased recharging of ATP. That gives us more energy for powerful muscular contractions used in short-term activities lasting from 5 to 10 seconds and, to a lesser degree, activities lasting up to 30 seconds and beyond. So the extra creatine translates into greater power and strength by recharging ATP levels in the muscle cells, delaying fatigue and giving a quicker recovery from physical exertion.

In sports where there are bouts of intense activity separated by short rest periods, creatine can be very effective in helping to maintain peak power output. In training, creatine will allow athletes to work harder and longer, and that can make them stronger. The creatine increases muscle mass, which is beneficial in many sports, and by doing that it may also help reduce the incidence of injury. Creatine may also prevent or reduce the severity of traumatic brain injury, which is common in sports like boxing, football, ice hockey, skiing, snowboarding, and soccer. Creatine can also be used to help athletes rehabilitate from injuries more quickly, which can be of tremendous value in returning to competition as soon as possible.

Q: What other sports/physical activities can be helped by creatine?
A: Theoretically, creatine should help with the discus throw, the shot put, the javelin, and other throwing sports. It should also be somewhat effective with sports like soccer, which is largely aerobic, but involves anaerobic activity like short sprints and goal kicks. A study by Cox and associates published in 2002 found some performance enhancement in female soccer players in a simulated match play.

Q: What about basketball?
A: The same applies to basketball, which is largely aerobic, with all its running, but also has anaerobic aspects like jumping and "muscling" past an opponent.

Q: Does creatine work the same way in men and women or is there a difference in the benefits?
A: The studies on this are conflicting. A 2000 study published in the *International Journal of Sports Nutrition and Exercise Metabolism,* which focused on cycling power and hand grip strength, found that there was no difference between men and women in their response to creatine—both benefited.

Another study found that both men and women gained fat-free mass with creatine, but women did so to a lesser degree than men. So it appears that women benefit from creatine, but possibly not to the same extent as men. However, many more studies need to be done before we know all the facts. As is often the case with scientific studies, most of the creatine studies have been done using male subjects.

Q: *What do official sports organizations say about the use of creatine? Do any of them endorse it, say it is safe, discourage its use, or ban it?*
A: While many official sports organizations have policies against such dangerous muscle-building compounds as anabolic steroids (see Chapter Ten), there is almost nothing said about creatine. We can conclude that they do not see it as dangerous in any way—which apparently it is not—and that they do not object to its use.

One organization that has issued a statement is The American College of Sports Medicine (ACSM), which presented a position paper on creatine supplementation in 1998. The ACSM deals with the application of sports and exercise medicine and its members are physicians, trainers, and sports professionals.

Q: *What did the ACSM study say?*
A: The ACSM reviewed many studies on creatine and came to the conclusion that these studies had clearly shown that a regimen of creatine supplementation significantly enhances accumulation of creatine and creatine phosphate in skeletal muscle. The paper went on to say that creatine can improve recovery time between bouts of exercise; increase energy during intense intermittent activities; and benefit athletes participating in sports or activities that are short-term, intense bouts of exercise.

The paper said that short-term cycling, sprinting, jumping, and weight lifting could all benefit from supplemental creatine, while long-term cycling, swimming, and running would benefit little or not at all. Finally, the paper concluded that much more research is needed before we have all the information on creatine's benefits and drawbacks and exactly how it works.

Q: Have any government agencies made statements on creatine?
A: Yes. The U.S. Food and Drug Administration (FDA) advised athletes to consult physicians or health care professionals before embarking on any scheme of creatine loading or supplementation.

Q: Do you go along with that advice?
A: Yes, I do to some degree. But the fact is that most people do not consult health care professionals before taking nonprescription supplements. They buy and take vitamins without knowing the quality of the vitamins, whether they really need them, or if they might even be harmful to specific individuals.

So I would like to see people tested for their individual needs, and advised and monitored by a knowledgeable professional to be certain they are taking what they need, taking it the right way, and getting the best possible results.

Q: Do most medical doctors have the required knowledge to do this?
A: No, most of them do not. That's why "health care professional" is a better term. When it comes to using creatine, it can mean your nutritionist, coach, athletic trainer, or any other professional with sufficient training, knowledge, and experience to be able to help you.

Points to Remember

- Aerobic exercise requires oxygen and involves long-term, steady, low-intensity energy in activities such as long-distance running, swimming, bicycling, jogging, and walking.
- Anaerobic exercise does not require oxygen and involves short-term bursts of high-intensity energy in activities such as weight lifting, wrestling, football, and sprinting.

- Some activities, like basketball and soccer, combine aerobic and anaerobic exercise.
- Anaerobic activities benefit most from creatine supplements.
- Aspects of aerobic exercise, such as a last-minute sprint to end a race, may benefit from creatine.
- Weight gain caused by creatine can be a detriment to some athletes, like runners and jumpers, who may not be able to perform as well due to the added poundage.
- Studies comparing the benefits of creatine in men and women are few in number and conflicting. Some find equal benefits for men and women, while others find men achieving better results. More studies are needed in this area.
- Most official sports organizations do not have a position on creatine. However, The American College of Sports Medicine has found benefits from creatine supplementation and the FDA advises that athletes who use creatine supplements be monitored by health care professionals.

CHAPTER SEVEN

Selecting the Right Creatine Product

WHEN YOU GO to the health food store, you may be over-whelmed by the wide variety of creatine products. There are powders, liquids, gels, and candy bars, as well as products that combine creatine with many other ingredients. As a result, it can be very difficult to select the best product for your individual needs. In this chapter, we will talk about whether all creatine products are the same; the different forms of creatine that are available; what to look for on the product label; how to get more information from the manufacturer; how much to spend for your product; whether creatine products are government regulated; what impurities can be found in creatine supplements; and how you can be assured of product safety.

Q: Are all creatine products basically the same?
A: No, they are not.

Q: So if you go to a store and see cans of creatine powder made by different manufacturers, they are not necessarily the same product?

A: That's right. You have to know something about them in order to select the one that is best for you.

Q: In addition to different manufacturers, creatine is also available in many different forms. Do they also have important differences?
A: Yes, they can. As you say, creatine is available in many different forms or delivery systems. You can take creatine monohydrate, the most common form which is used in almost all the studies, and if you compare powders from different companies, they will not all be the same. Many will be similar, but some may be of inferior quality or have a lower concentration of the actual creatine in the product.

Q: Who makes the creatine in these products?
A: Surprisingly, there are only a few manufacturers in the world and all the different companies that sell creatine obtain it from these sources. Basically, almost all the creatine we purchase is manufactured either in the United States, Germany, Norway, or China.

Q: What are the main differences among these manufacturers?
A: Scientific analyses have shown that the creatine from the United States, Germany and Norway is superior to the creatine from China, which is often of poor quality and has more contaminants.

Q: How can consumers know the source of the creatine in the product they buy?
A: Some products contain the name or logo ("Creapure") of the German manufacturer, Degussa, which has a patent on its creatine manufacturing process. But in most cases, consumers cannot learn the creatine source from the product label. You can try to contact the manufacturer and ask for this information and reputable companies will provide it.

Q: What is actually in the creatine?
A: In the past when it was first used as a supplement, creatine was extracted from meat. Today, the creatine you buy is a synthetic product, usually made from cyanamide, water, and sodium sarcosinate. This is a much less expensive way to produce it. Powdered creatine monohydrate should be 100 percent creatine monohydrate, which is creatine bound to water. In reality, some products may have more than 5 percent impurities.

Q: What are some of the contaminants that have been found in creatine products?
A: There are quite a few, including creatinine (the body's waste byproduct of creatine which is excreted in urine), dicyandiamide (a derivative of one of the chemicals used in creatine production which is used in production of fertilizers and explosives), thiourea (a suspected carcinogen), dihydrotriazines (a byproduct of creatine production whose safety is currently unknown) and even detectable amounts of mercury and lead, which are most commonly found in creatine products coming from China. Chinese creatine, by the way, is less expensive than the American or German products and is more likely to be found in low-cost creatine products.

Q: Are these contaminants dangerous?
A: Not every contaminant has been tested for safety, so it's a good idea to avoid them if possible. Beyond safety, these impurities are a waste of money. You buy creatine for performance enhancement—contaminants do not help build your strength and muscle.

Q: How can you know if you are purchasing a product that has few or no contaminants?
A: One way is to buy products made by the big companies, the

ones that advertise widely and are known for quality. If you buy a non-brand name or a product that is much less expensive than the others, your chances of getting a contaminated product are much greater. That doesn't mean that all such products are bad. We are just talking about the odds if you have no further information.

Q: How can you get that information?
A: You can try by contacting the company directly, whether through the internet, on the phone, or by mail. Ask for documentation on the contents of their product and where the product was made and by whom. Reputable companies will almost always provide such information to consumers.

Q: What specific information should you look for?
A: One of the things you should ask for is a laboratory assay, an analysis of what is in the product, especially if it is from an independent laboratory, rather than from the company itself. Some of the things an assay can check are the purity of the product and how much creatine is actually in it.

You can also have a creatine product analyzed by an independent laboratory on your own. Although I have not done this with creatine, I have had other supplements checked out. One product that was analyzed turned out to contain 0 percent of one of the ingredients listed on the label!

Q: How are creatine products analyzed?
A: One of the methods that should be used is high-performance liquid chromatography (HPLC), which is a reliable method of determination. Creatine can also be assayed for toxins such as heavy metals, for microbes or bacteria and for some of the more common impurities in creatine that we already mentioned.

Q: What if the company does not send you this kind of assay report?
A: If they don't send an independent assay, you may want to look for a different product. Also if they send you an assay that only checks for one or two items, that might be a cause of concern, as well.

Q: So a good creatine manufacturer will send you a detailed independent assay, is that right?
A: Yes, I think that is a safe assumption.

Q: In what different forms can creatine be purchased?
A: You can buy creatine phosphate, which is the form that is found in the body, but it is expensive and not worth the money. Creatine citrate is another form which may be more soluble than creatine monohydrate, but that is not yet supported by research. Creatine monohydrate is the form that is found in almost all creatine supplements and that has been used in almost all creatine studies.

Creatine monohydrate is also available in micronized form, which means that the particle size is smaller, so that theoretically, it can be better absorbed by the intestinal tract. But regular creatine monohydrate appears to be absorbed very efficiently, so a more expensive micronized product may not be worth the money.

There is also effervescent creatine powder, but I don't know of any published studies proving that this form is more effective. In addition to the most commonly used form, which is creatine monohydrate powder, you can also find creatine in liquids, gels, capsules, chewable tablets, bars, and chewing gum.

Q: What about the amount of creatine that you get in these different products? Is it the same?
A: It could be the same, but you have to read the labels. The

average creatine dose is 2 to 5 grams and that could be available in a candy bar. But the form of a candy bar might not be the most efficient way to take creatine. You could be getting other ingredients you don't want or need, such as artificial flavors and colors, and you may not be getting the liquid you need for optimal absorption when you take creatine. So I generally recommend the powder form for most people.

Q: *Is liquid creatine an effective form?*
A: From the research I've seen, the liquid form of creatine is unstable and not effective. The creatine converts to creatinine very rapidly in the bottle, even before you've purchased the product.

Q: *Why is that a problem?*
A: Because you're taking creatine supplements in order to get actual creatine into your body. The action of the creatine has to take place within your cells for you to get the energy- and muscle-boosting benefits. Once creatine converts to creatinine, it becomes a waste product, and your body will excrete it. So there is no point in buying creatine that has converted to creatinine. Creatinine does nothing for strength or muscle building.

Q: *Have studies shown that liquid creatine is less effective than the powder form?*
A: There is a study involving assays of liquid creatine done at three different laboratories that showed it contained only 10 milligrams of creatine per serving, when the label claimed it contained 250 times that amount. It is possible that when the product was manufactured that was true, but the combination of creatine with the liquid ingredients resulted in far less actual creatine once the product was ready to be consumed.

Another study published in 2002 in the *Journal of*

Pharmaceutical Biomedicine concluded that "some of the over-the-counter products tested contained a very low level of creatine in contrast to their label claim. Substantial conversion of creatine into creatinine was noticed in liquid formulation."

I have also seen advertisements for liquid creatine that present information about the efficacy and safety of powdered crea-

---

Adam: Don't Expect Miracles

A 44-year-old account executive, Adam never liked his skinny body. He consulted me about how he could become more muscular. I did an assessment and gave him advice on how to change his diet and use weight training and creatine supplements. Since he had never exercised regularly before, this program meant a lot of changes for Adam.

He began going to the gym six days a week and following the exercise program I had outlined for him. Adam also changed his diet and began using a formula containing creatine, carbohydrates, glutamine, taurine, sodium, and magnesium phosphate. When Adam called me two weeks later, he was concerned about his progress. He told me that he had gained only three pounds and even though his strength was improving, he felt discouraged.

I told Adam that I thought he was doing very well, and he should stick to his program. Although he had expected to gain more weight after two weeks, I explained that his weight gain was fine for him and if he continued, he would gain more in the future. I cautioned him not to expect overnight miracles. Adam responded that he was doing so much hard work that he thought the results should be a lot better. Going to the gym so often, working so hard, and keeping up with his eating plan were a lot of trouble and he wasn't sure it was worth it. When Adam failed to show up for his next appointment, I could only assume that his impatience had led to a decision that the healthy eating, weight training, and creatine were not what he wanted. Perhaps he will be back one day.

tine monohydrate that is simply untrue. These kinds of ads can spread false information to people who use creatine and convince them that liquid creatine is superior in some way, which to the best of my knowledge, it is not.

So my conclusion is not to use creatine in liquid form until manufacturers solve the problems of the creatine breaking down in the bottle prior to consumption.

Q: *Is it better to buy pure creatine or creatine that is combined with other substances?*
A: Most of the studies on creatine involve creatine alone, not other substances. But there is also some research showing that certain other compounds may be beneficial when combined with creatine. For instance, a 1996 study indicated that ingesting carbohydrates half an hour after creatine increases muscle creatine levels by 60 percent over using plain creatine.

Q: *Are there creatine products that combine it with carbohydrates?*
A: Yes. For example, you can find dextrose, maltose, potato starch and glucose polymers in some creatine products. You can also find creatine products that have added ingredients, including protein, taurine, sodium, and others (see Chapter Ten). The idea is that these other ingredients help to increase creatine transport into the cells. While there is little potential for benefit in attempting to enhance intestinal absorption of creatine, maximizing transport from the blood into the cells can really improve results from using creatine.

Q: *But you will be paying more for these products with added ingredients?*
A: Yes, you will.

Q: Does combining creatine with carbohydrates make the creatine more efficient?
A: Using enough of the right type of carbohydrate at the right time significantly increases muscle creatine levels. The aforementioned 1996 study compared creatine loading (5 grams four times a day) with and without carbohydrates. The carbohydrates were simple sugars in solution at a very large dose of 93 grams. This sugar solution was ingested half an hour after each creatine dose.

The reason for the delay in drinking the sugar solution is that whereas creatine levels in the blood peak an hour after ingestion, insulin levels peak about half an hour after drinking a sugar solution. It is important for creatine and insulin levels to peak simultaneously for optimal insulin-mediated transport of creatine into muscle cells.

A 1998 study found that it takes a large amount of insulin to produce an increase in muscle creatine levels. This study confirmed that sugar solutions containing much less than the amount used in the 1996 study would not likely be helpful. Based on this research, using carbohydrate to increase muscle creatine levels requires ingestion of close to 100 grams of simple carbohydrate (dextrose or maltose, for example) thirty minutes after taking creatine.

Despite these studies, I still have some reservations about using high carbohydrates with creatine. For a lot of people who have problems with carbohydrate metabolism, excess carbohydrates are not a good idea. That is probably a less immediate health problem for young, lean active athletes, but for a lot of Americans, consuming a high level of carbohydrates with the goal of increasing your insulin levels is not beneficial.

Q: Why can that be a problem?
A: Because high carbohydrate consumption and consequent

high blood glucose and insulin levels are associated with a lot of negative health effects, including weight gain around the mid-section, excess fat storage in general, high blood pressure, high cholesterol and triglycerides, diabetes, increased risk of cardio-vascular disease, damage to body tissues and accelerated biological aging, to name a few.

Q: Then what would you recommend for the average consumer who wants to purchase and use creatine in the most effective way?
A: Each individual must make a value judgment. How much effort and expense are you willing to put out for optimal creatine effectiveness?

I think the best way to load with creatine is by following each creatine dose half an hour later with about 50 grams of whey protein and 50 grams of simple carbohydrate. A 2000 study found that a mixture of 50 grams of protein and 47 grams of carbohydrate were as effective as 96 grams of carbohydrate in raising blood insulin levels and enhancing muscle creatine concentrations.

It is possible that you could get a similar effect from a lesser amount of carbohydrate and protein if other insulin stimulators, mimics and sensitizers are simultaneously supplemented.

Q: Then you are in favor of combining protein and carbohydrates with your creatine intake?
A: I favor the protein-carbohydrate mixture because it does not raise blood sugar levels as much as the pure carbohydrate drink. The protein-carbohydrate drink also contains 12.5 grams of fat, 450 milligrams of sodium, 750 milligrams of potassium, about 675 milligrams of chloride, 750 milligrams of calcium, 300 milligrams of magnesium, 500 milligrams of phosphorus, and 15 milligrams of iron.

Q: Why should people consider taking creatine along with these other ingredients?
A: Because it is possible that there may be a beneficial effect from some of these other ingredients. For example, a study comparing 5.25 grams of creatine monohydrate and 1 gram of glucose, with 5.25 grams of creatine monohydrate and 33 grams of glucose, 633 milligrams of sodium and potassium phosphate, and 1 gram of taurine found the latter combination produced greater gains in fat-free mass, strength, vertical jump, and 100-yard dash time.

Q: Should you buy creatine with the other ingredients already mixed in or should you take them separately, and if so, when?
A: Ideally, the formula of additional ingredients should be consumed half an hour after taking creatine. A compromise is to take a formula containing all these ingredients at once. Some manufacturers are trying to deal with this issue by using a blend of three different carbohydrates designed to raise blood sugar and insulin at different rates. But I am not aware of any published research on these blends.

One study found that after just one day of creatine loading, the effectiveness of carbohydrate and protein in augmenting creatine transport was dropping. So a question remains: how long does one need to take creatine with protein and carbohydrate? Perhaps not beyond the loading phase—we don't know at this point.

Q: What is your general advice about buying creatine products that have additional ingredients?
A: If you don't mind the added expense and you want to try some of the other compounds with creatine, they appear to be safe and can be effective in helping the creatine to work and in building muscle. I recommend looking for a product that has carbohy-

drate, some protein, alpha lipoic acid, taurine, sodium and potassium phosphates, D-pinitol, or some combination of these ingredients. All of them have some research to support them. I think
many people could also benefit from adding glutamine, magnesium, arginine, and 4-hydroxyisoleucine.

Q: *Is it easy to find such products?*
A: Usually it is, but it might take a little searching. Some of these
ingredients are widely used with creatine, but others, like alpha
lipoic acid, may be in only one product because of patent protection.

Q: *Are there any ingredients you should avoid?*
A: Yes, as I've already mentioned, I think you should avoid artificial flavors and colors, which you certainly do not need and
which could have potential adverse effects on some people.

Q: *Do different people need different creatine products? If so,
how do you know which one is right for you?*
A: People are biochemically unique, so no single product is best
for everyone. The only way to find out is to work with a health
care professional to try to determine which product best suits
your individual needs.

Q: *What specific kinds of things can you find out by working
with a health care professional?*
A: For example, people who have certain health conditions, such
as diabetes, hypoglycemia, obesity, high cholesterol or triglycerides, or high blood pressure, should be wary of formulas with
a lot of carbohydrate. And there are other people who have kidney or liver problems who need to use caution with creatine and
who should not use products with too much protein.

Then, there are people who can benefit from, but need to be
cautious with the insulin sensitizers, alpha lipoic acid, chromium

and D-pinitol. People with diabetes, for instance, may have a lowering of their blood sugar, which needs to be controlled. If they are on medication, they may need to reduce their medication in conjunction with consulting a doctor in order to use these creatine products safely. Anyone using creatine for its benefits on brain health should consider using it with alpha lipoic acid, which is good for brain health in its own right. (See Chapter Nine for more information on who should not use creatine and who should be cautious.)

Q: How much should creatine cost? Are more expensive products better?
A: It's not that simple. You can spend a lot and get an inferior product and you can spend less and get an excellent product. So price is no guarantee of what you are getting, but price can be a general gauge.

A very inexpensive product may well be of inferior quality, as we have often seen with some of the creatine manufactured in China. And very expensive products may contain additives you don't really need or may just be overpriced in order to maximize profits for the company.

Q: Does the form of creatine also influence price?
A: Definitely. I don't recommend liquid creatine because of the instability already mentioned, but in addition, gram for gram, the amount of creatine you get in liquid products makes it much more expensive. The same is true of creatine in capsule or tablet forms. Whenever a compound is put into a capsule or pill, the cost goes up. So if you are really set on taking creatine in these forms, you have to be prepared to pay more for it.

Q: So a product in the form of pure creatine monohydrate powder is the best value for your money?

A: That's right. Anything that requires further processing will usually add to the cost of the creatine.

Q: What about size?
A: That also affects price and as with most products, you can almost always save money on creatine by buying it in larger sizes. So if you plan to be using creatine for a while, it is more economical to buy a larger size.

Q: Approximately how much should consumers pay for their creatine supplements?
A: Of course, prices vary according to the manufacturer, the store, the location, and so on. But we can say that a pound of plain creatine monohydrate powder should cost between $15 and $50.

Q: Where can people buy it?
A: Today, many people shop online for their supplements and if you know what you want, it can be a way to save money. There's also the convenience of not having to go out to a store and buy it. But most people still buy creatine in their local health food store. It's such a popular supplement, that you can also often find it in some larger supermarkets, drug stores, health clubs, and gyms. You can also buy from a licensed nutritionist. If you stick with a big company and buy in the form of creatine monohydrate powder, you should be safe no matter where you choose to buy your product.

Q: What government agencies regulate creatine products? Do they assure product purity and safety?
A: The Food and Drug Administration (FDA) is involved in the regulation of nutritional products—but only superficially. They don't get very involved unless there is a serious cause for concern about a product being dangerous and unsafe to consumers.

So no, there are no governmental agencies working to assure the complete safety, purity, or potency of creatine products. In fact, it has been discovered through independent tests that there are nutritional supplements on the shelves of various stores that have very little or even none of the active ingredients they claim to have on their labels! So it's important to realize that there is no guarantee about what you are getting when you buy these largely unregulated products. Some companies are very good at packaging, marketing and making their products look and sound very good, but that is no guarantee that they are what they claim to be or that they will help you in any way.

Q: What should people do about this situation?
A: Consumers have to protect themselves by remaining well informed about what they are buying.

Q: Do you think there should be stricter regulations about nutritional supplements and products?
A: It might be a good idea, but the FDA does not have the manpower or budget to take on the huge task of regulating the nutritional supplement industry. On the positive side, however, there is a lot of self-regulation in the industry. There are certain accepted manufacturing procedures and some companies voluntarily invite the FDA to come in and inspect their labs and plants. In that way, they get an independent overview, perhaps make some improvements, and let customers know this has been done in order to increase confidence that they are producing safe products.

Q: What is your overall view of creatine products?
A: I believe most of them are safe and if you are careful about what you buy and follow some of the guidelines in this book, you should be able to easily find an effective creatine product that will work well for you.

Points to Remember

• All creatine products are not the same.

• The form of the creatine product—powder, liquid, gel, candy bar, etc.— can affect the quality and potency of the creatine.

• Only a few countries manufacture creatine and one of them, China, has been known to produce inferior creatine in the past.

• When buying creatine, it is usually safer to stick to well-known brands.

• You should request product information, including independent laboratory test analysis results, from the company. Most reputable companies will provide them to customers.

• Many creatine products have been found to contain contaminants. Although they are not generally considered harmful, it is best to avoid them.

• Pure creatine monohydrate powder is the form most often used, most tested, and most economical.

• Liquid creatine is generally unstable and degrades in the bottle prior to use, so it is not a recommended form.

• For most people, combining creatine with carbohydrates and protein can increase muscle cell creatine levels and thus, overall results.

• No governmental agencies regulate creatine products, so consumers must do their own research to find the purest and most effective creatine product.

CHAPTER EIGHT

How Do You Use Creatine?

THERE'S A BIT more to creatine than just mixing it up with some liquid and drinking it. In fact, there's quite a lot to know. In this chapter, you will learn about "loading" and "cycling" and how to decide if they are right for you; how much creatine you should take for your individual needs; whether to combine creatine with other substances for maximum benefits; whether other foods have an adverse effect on creatine's action; and what to do if creatine doesn't seem to work for you.

Q: Why is it important to check with your health care professional before taking creatine?
A: There are a few reasons why it's always a good idea to consult a health care professional before taking creatine. One of the most important is that you could have a health condition that would make creatine supplementation more of a concern (see Chapter Nine). Or you might be on a medication that has an effect on kidney or liver function and which could, therefore, interfere with creatine metabolism. Or you might have a condition or be on a

medication that would reduce creatine's effectiveness. Also, you might have a condition that would influence what supplements you should or should not take along with creatine. Finally, if your health care professional is knowledgeable about creatine, you could get some good advice about how to use it most effectively.

Q: Can you explain the term "loading" in regard to the use of creatine supplements?
A: Loading refers to starting off with a very high dose of creatine for a short period of time in order to really saturate the muscles and get a quicker effect. The typical loading phase involves 5 grams of creatine taken four times a day for five to seven days. That regimen usually increases muscle creatine levels by about 25 percent. So loading is a good way to get rapid results from creatine supplementation.

Q: You use the loading phase when you first start taking creatine, is that right?
A: Yes.

Q: What if you haven't taken it for a while? Do you use a loading phase again?
A: It's usually a good idea to use a loading phase if you haven't taken creatine for a while. It may be somewhat inconvenient to have to take it this way, but it's definitely the best way to get quick results.

Q: Should everyone use a loading phase? If not, who should use it and who should not, or is it just an individual choice?
A: If you want to see quick results, use a loading phase. If you're patient or if you don't want to be inconvenienced by having to use creatine four times a day, an alternative approach is to just use the maintenance dose.

Q: What is a maintenance dose?
A: One study found that using 3 grams of creatine a day for twenty-eight days resulted in the same tissue levels of creatine as using a loading phase first and then going into a maintenance phase. In other words, the end results were the same, but the people using loading got the creatine into their muscle cells more rapidly. Importantly, 3 grams seems to be the minimum effective dose for most individuals. Another study found 2 grams of creatine daily for six weeks to be ineffective.

Q: Are there any people who should not use a loading phase?
A: People who have kidney or liver problems or are on certain medications may be advised by their health care professionals not to use loading but to use creatine on a maintenance dose from the beginning to avoid any impact on kidney or liver function by taking in too much creatine at one time.

Q: What does the term "cycling" mean in regard to creatine supplementation?
A: Cycling refers to using creatine for a period of time, then discontinuing use for a while, and then starting to use creatine again. The concept of cycling really comes from the use of anabolic steroids. Because steroids have toxic effects on the body, people have used cycling in order to minimize their dangers. So they will use steroids for a period of time and then stop in order to allow their bodies to detoxify and heal to a certain extent. Then they will go back on the steroids. But with steroids, unlike creatine, you have a very dangerous substance that should not be used at all (see Chapter Ten).

Q: How does cycling work for creatine?
A: Because creatine is so safe, it is not necessary to cycle it for health reasons. Some people have a concern that using creatine

supplements will reduce the body's ability to manufacture its own internal creatine, so certain people may decide to cycle for that reason. I personally think it is unlikely that using creatine regularly will cause any trouble because we ingest creatine in food all the time, especially if we eat meat and fish. Studies have found that even though the body may produce less creatine when a person's intake of supplements is greater than usual, as soon as the creatine intake is lowered, the body produces more. So I don't see any evidence that it is dangerous to your health to take creatine without cycling.

Q: *What about creatine's effectiveness? Can cycling improve it in any way?*
A: There are people who believe that cycling may enhance the effectiveness of creatine. First you use creatine for a period of time, and you then discontinue its use, letting the creatine levels in your muscles decrease to some degree. Then after awhile, you go through another loading phase. There is some belief that by doing this, you can raise your creatine levels to a higher level than they were before the cycling.

Q: *How long do you have to discontinue using creatine for these effects to take place?*
A: When you stop using creatine, it takes about four weeks for muscle creatine levels to return to their pre-supplementation levels. But if you want to cycle creatine to try to get better results, you should discontinue it for two to three weeks and then go through another loading phase.

Q: *What does discontinuing creatine actually to?*
A: Discontinuing creatine may increase the activity of creatine transporter proteins in the body. High levels of creatine outside the cells stimulate production of a protein that inactivates the

creatine transporter. So if you cycle and discontinue creatine for a period of time, then the transporters may become more active. Then, when you load the creatine, you can theoretically get more into your cells.

Q: You say "theoretically." Does that mean there is no definitive scientific evidence that this actually happens?
A: That's right. But it is something that people using creatine have experimented with and that some people find effective. So I advise people to try it and see if it works for them.

Q: Exactly what should they do?
A: I suggest that prior to a competition or whenever you want to have the maximum benefits of creatine, cycle it and go through another loading phase. Of course, it may be wise to experiment with this when there is less pressure for results, such as during the off-season.

Q: How do you determine exactly how much creatine to use?
A: When it comes to exact individual needs, it can be guess work. But there are certain guidelines you can use. For instance, if you are bigger, have more muscle mass or are involved in heavy strength training, you usually need more creatine. Your individual diet can also increase your need for creatine; for example, if it is low in meat and fish, the foods with the highest creatine content.

Q: Are there any tests to determine your body's creatine level?
A: At this time, there are no readily available direct ways of assessing your creatine status. Most people don't want to undergo a muscle biopsy with a needle, and special tests using phosphorus 31 NMR spectroscopy are expensive and not readily available. Blood and urine tests are available for creatinine (the

breakdown product of creatine). The balance of creatinine and certain other biochemicals can give you a rough indication of your creatine status, but this is an imprecise indicator and probably not worth the effort. It is best just to try creatine and see how you respond.

Q: What are creatine recommendations for the average person?
A: The protocol that has been used in many studies is a loading phase of 5 grams of creatine four times a day for five to seven days, followed by a maintenance dose of 3 to 5 grams a day. For a large person with a heavy exercise routine, 5 grams a day to as much as 10 grams a day may be needed.

There is also a formula recommended by one researcher that is based on body weight. Take .3 grams of creatine per kilogram of body weight for the loading phase for five days and then take one-tenth of that amount for the maintenance phase.

Q: How many pounds are equivalent to a kilogram of body weight?
A: A kilogram is roughly 2.2 pounds.

Q: What is the best way to take creatine? You have recommended the powdered form, so what should you mix it with?
A: Depending on your individual needs, you should take about 5 grams of creatine powder mixed with about 8 or more ounces of juice or water. Sixteen ounces of grape juice supplies a good dose (close to 80 grams) of carbohydrate. I recommend grape juice because of its carbohydrate makeup, which includes dextrose. Dextrose appears to be a good transporter for creatine, as opposed to some of the other fruit juices. But you can mix your creatine powder with water if you want to. Early studies mixed creatine with hot coffee or tea, but juice or another carbohydrate beverage is preferable.

If your goal is weight gain, take creatine with a lot of carbohydrate and protein. Overall, my preference is to take creatine with, or ideally thirty minutes before, a mixture of 50 grams of simple carbohydrate and 50 grams of protein (preferably whey). Many companies make protein and carbohydrate powders, which can be mixed with water. You can also buy creatine formulas containing protein and carbohydrate.

Q: If you are using pure creatine powder, how does it taste?
A: Plain creatine monohydrate powder should have no taste.

Q: When is the best time to take creatine—before, with or after meals?
A: Research has not answered that question. I can speculate that, based on results of carbohydrate and protein feedings with creatine, prior to meals may be best. Creatine transport into muscle cells may be optimized when creatine is taken thirty minutes before a meal because of the insulin release caused by many foods.

Q: For the best results, should you combine creatine with other nutrients, such as vitamins, minerals, or amino acids?
A: For the best results, creatine experts advise combining creatine with carbohydrates. As we have just recommended, you can use about 50 grams of carbohydrates and 50 grams of protein for maximal effect. There are studies showing that carbohydrate and protein combined with creatine supplements are more effective in transporting creatine into the cells. I also think it's better for health purposes to use a mixture of carbohydrate and protein, rather than 95 or 100 grams of plain carbohydrate.

Q: What other helpful substances can be combined with creatine?
A: Studies indicate that taurine, sodium, alpha lipoic acid, and

Janet: Creatine for Optimal Health

A 63-year-old attorney, Janet consulted me for weight loss, general health improvement, and disease prevention. Janet had quite a few health issues, including osteopenia or low bone density, which is a mild form of osteoporosis; elevated blood cholesterol and triglycerides; excess body fat, especially around the midsection; carbohydrate cravings; fatigue and weakness; irritability; insomnia; and a poor memory. She also had a family history of type 2 diabetes, heart disease, and Alzheimer's disease.

I examined Janet's current health problems, along with her personal and family health history and found a pattern, a common link. The link was insulin resistance, or impaired carbohydrate metabolism.

When muscle and fat cells don't respond efficiently to insulin's signals, a variety of serious adverse changes occur in different aspects of metabolism. Increased abdominal body fat and high levels of blood triglycerides and cholesterol are all consistent with insulin resistance. While insulin resistance is not the only cause of these symptoms, it is still a very common and powerful one, affecting about one out of every three Americans. And further laboratory testing showed that Janet was, in fact, insulin resistant.

I measured Janet's body composition and found that her body fat was high and her body cell mass low. An important measure, body cell mass is the tissue that does most of the metabolic work and calorie burning. Janet's body was in a declining state, with weakened muscles and an acceleration of the aging process.

I developed a diet and lifestyle program for Janet designed to improve her metabolism and help her get healthier. For the first time in her life, Janet began weight training, and she also continued with the treadmill exercise she had been doing. I prescribed an improved diet, along with nutritional supplements and creatine monohydrate.

I recommended creatine for Janet to help increase her body cell mass and intracellular water, normalize carbohydrate metabolism, lower bad cholesterol and triglycerides, improve energy and strength and protect her brain cells from damage (as occurs with Alzheimer's disease).

Because Janet's cells were not responding efficiently to insulin's signals, I decided not to have her take creatine with a high glycemic index drink, which would raise blood sugar and insulin levels dramatically. Instead, I told her to mix the creatine with a shake designed to improve the cells' sensitivity to insulin. Among other ingredients, this shake contains chromium, alpha lipoic acid, magnesium, inositol, vanadyl sulfate, biotin, soluble fibers, isoflavones, and vitamin E.

The program worked very well for Janet and after only three months, she looked and felt much better. She had lost four pounds, including seven pounds of fat; she had gained three pounds of muscle, lost two inches from her waistline, and her body cell mass and intracellular water levels were both healthier. Her total cholesterol dropped by 22 percent and triglycerides by 35 percent. Janet reported that her energy was now much higher and her other symptoms much improved. Janet is continuing with her program, cycling creatine on for two months and off for one.

D-pinitol can all help with creatine transport. A newer formulation by one company contains 4-hydroxyisoleucine, which although not proven to increase creatine transport, should theoretically do so because of the effect of 4-hydroxyisoleucine on stimulating sugar-induced insulin secretion and possibly muscle cell insulin sensitivity.

This compound may, like protein, reduce the amount of sugar necessary to cause a creatine-enhancing insulin spike.

Q: Are there specific substances that can help creatine increase muscle growth?

A: Yes, there are ways to provide synergistic effects on muscle growth, such as using glutamine or HMB (beta-hydroxy-beta-methylbutyrate) (see Chapter Ten). For instance, one 2001 study by Jowko and associates, which appeared in *Nutrition*, studied forty subjects over a three-week period, giving the first group a placebo, the second group creatine, the third group HMB, and the fourth group a combination of creatine and HMB. Over three weeks of resistance training, all the subjects gained lean body mass, but the groups taking creatine, HMB, and the combination of creatine and HMB gained more than the placebo group. And it was the group taking the combination of creatine and HMB that gained the most. So at least according to this study, combining creatine with HMB can give better results.

Q: Some creatine supplements include other ingredients, such as carbohydrate, sodium, protein, HMB or glutamine in their product. If you use pure creatine powder, can you add the other ingredients yourself in the form of separate supplements and get the same results?
A: Yes, of course you can. I don't know if there are any creatine products that include all these ingredients—you will have to check that out for yourself. But I think the most important ones are carbohydrate, protein, sodium, and taurine. The insulin sensitizers, alpha lipoic acid, D-pinitol, 4-hydroxyisoleucine and magnesium, also appear to be valuable. Additional arginine and glutamine may also be helpful.

Q: Does caffeine have an adverse effect on creatine? If so, why? Should people using creatine to build muscle give up caffeine?
A: There are several studies that indicate that caffeine has a negative effect on the performance enhancement of creatine. The reasons for this are not yet clear. But as we have seen, early creatine studies dissolved the powder in caffeinated beverages and

it still had performance-enhancing effects. Therefore, it is possible that caffeine may have a minor negative effect for some people and be fine for others.

So while you may get a better result using creatine without consuming caffeine, you don't have to give it up altogether if you don't want to. I have personally seen coffee drinkers respond well to creatine supplements. It's really an individual matter and each person can observe his or her response to creatine with and without caffeine. Finally, I think moderation is important, so if you use caffeine, try not to use too much.

Q: Is there a preferred time of day to take creatine?
A: Studies have not shown that any specific time of day is best. It's more important to take creatine consistently. If you miss one day, that won't affect your creatine stores too much, but if you miss several days or take it sporadically, it will not work as well.

The best time to take creatine is after workouts, because that's when you will have increased creatine uptake by the muscle cells, increased formation of glycogen and increased protein synthesis for building muscles.

Q: If you don't work out every day, should you still take it at the same time every day?
A: It's a good idea to do that because then you won't forget to take it and your body will also be ingesting the same amount on a daily basis, which will help to maintain a consistent amount in your cells.

Q: Is it better to take your maintenance dose of creatine at one time or divided throughout the day?
A: That has not yet been determined. Some experts believe it's beneficial to take your maintenance dose at one time each day and others recommend dividing it into two or three doses during

the day. Again, it's something that individuals will have to determine for themselves by trial and error in order to find out what works best for them. If your maintenance dose is more than 5 grams, it should be taken in divided doses to minimize wasting it in the urine because muscle cells can't absorb more than a few grams at one time.

Q: *If creatine works so well, is more better? Can you take too much and if so, what happens if you do?*
A: No, more is not better. There is a limit to how much creatine your muscles can store and once your intake goes above that limit, your body will simply excrete the excess creatine in the urine. So yes, you can take too much and if you take too much at one time, you will not only be wasting the creatine, you may also get some gastrointestinal upset.

Q: *How much is too much?*
A: For almost everyone, more than 20 grams a day is excessive. If you want optimal results, go through the loading phase at 20 grams a day (divided into four separate doses of 5 grams each). When you do this, it appears that the creatine is most rapidly absorbed by the muscles in the first couple of days of the loading phase. So going through even five to seven days of loading may be excessive, although it is safe.

No need for more than 20 grams a day has ever been established, so if you take more, you will waste your money, inconvenience yourself and possibly experience some side effects, as well. Using more than 5 grams at one time is probably also excessive.

Q: *Is it necessary to combine creatine with exercise in order for it to work?*
A: No it isn't necessary, but the results are far better if you exer-

cise. Exercise increases creatine uptake into the muscles and of course, exercising your muscles is the most important thing you can do for muscle growth and performance. Remember that creatine is mainly an ergogenic aid, and it works in coordination with muscle contraction.

But if for some reason you are not able or willing to exercise, and you just want to experiment with creatine to see if it benefits you in any way, by all means, go ahead. You may have some good results. But those results will definitely be far superior with exercise as opposed to without it.

Q: What happens if creatine doesn't seem to work for you? Why would that happen?
A: There are times when creatine does not seem to work and there are individuals who do not seem to respond to creatine supplements.

When creatine supplementation fails to produce benefits, it is because cellular creatine and creatine phosphate levels have not increased sufficiently. After four to six days of creatine loading, increases in total muscle creatine concentration range from 5 to 30 percent, depending on the individual. That is a tremendous six-fold difference from person to person. It takes roughly a 20 percent increase in order to get performance-enhancing effects. People with the lowest initial muscle creatine concentrations will experience greater benefits and increases in creatine levels from supplementation.

So the most obvious reason for creatine not working is that your muscles' creatine levels are so high that the effect of supplementation is minimal. This is unlikely to be the case with vegetarians.

Another reason might be that you are not using the correct dosage of creatine and are taking less than your body requires. Not being consistent with creatine supplementation could be another reason for lack of response. Or perhaps you are using an inferior product and are not getting the amount of creatine that is on the label.

You could also have certain health problems that affect creatine transport. One of the most common is insulin resistance, where the body's cells do not respond to insulin signals effectively. You may also have a problem where your cells are not producing ATP properly and that could have an impact.

You might also have nutrient deficiencies or poor health, and that could make creatine less able to work effectively. Altered hormone status, such as a low level of insulin, norepinephrine, IGF-1 or T-3, the active thyroid hormone, could also cause a problem because they all stimulate muscle creatine accumulation.

Perhaps you are not using the creatine in combination with a carbohydrate and so it is not working at its full benefit. Importantly, a study found that when creatine was loaded along with a high carbohydrate solution, the average creatine accumulation shot up to 25 percent. If creatine is taken in this way, or with a combination carbohydrate-protein solution, almost everyone will respond.

Another reason for a poor response is that you may not be exercising, or not exercising enough to put the creatine to work. As we've just mentioned, caffeine may reduce creatine effectiveness. And finally, cell culture studies indicate that certain medications, such as beta blockers (atenolol, butoxamine, and propranolol), inhibit creatine uptake.

Q: What is the best type of exercise to activate creatine?
A: The right type of exercise is heavy resistance training, as in weight training. Don't forget that if you are not exercising or if you are not doing the appropriate exercise, you are not going to get the full benefits from creatine.

Q: If you use creatine supplementation, what typical results can you expect to achieve?
A: The average response to creatine supplementation is a 10 to 15 percent increase in strength and an additional 1–3 percent increase in lean body mass over one to three months of training.

Q: How long does it take for creatine to begin to work?
A: For most people, it takes about a day or more of loading with creatine for it to begin to have an effect.

The quickest published response that I am aware of is seventeen hours. In a 2002 double-blind placebo-controlled crossover study, five wrestlers took creatine with glucose or a glucose placebo after undergoing rapid weight loss. Their high intensity exercise capacity was measured before and after the weight loss. They then took a creatine or placebo drink during a seventeen-hour recovery period, at the end of which they underwent a third round of testing. It was found that the placebo did not change exercise work capacity, but the creatine supplement produced a 19.2 percent increase in high intensity work. So it looks like it can be beneficial for wrestlers to take creatine after weigh-in.

Q: What happens when you stop using creatine?
A: The muscle mass that you have worked so hard to build will remain for a while, especially if you continue to exercise and eat properly. You will probably lose a little in size and strength as your creatine stores return to pre-supplementation levels. That should take about a month. But overall, you will be stronger and more muscular than if you had never used creatine. And you can always go back to it in the future if you want to.

Points to Remember

- To safeguard your health, always consult a knowledgeable health care professional before taking creatine.
- Many people use a loading phase for creatine, initially taking larger amounts for a few days in order to get faster results.
- You can get the same overall results after a few weeks of using a lower, regular amount of creatine as you will by using a loading phase.
- Some people cycle creatine, taking it for a while, then stopping, and then resuming it later on. Some people believe that cycling helps to keep the body's internal creatine manufacturing process working well; others think cycling eventually increases creatine stores in the body.
- People need to experiment in order to find out if loading and cycling work well for them.
- Bigger and more active people usually need larger creatine doses than smaller, less active people.
- Creatine works best when combined with carbohydrates.
- Other nutrients, such as protein, sodium, taurine, alpha lipoic acid and others may increase creatine's effectiveness. Caffeine, especially in large amounts, may be a negative factor.
- For best effects, take creatine every day at the same time, whether in one dose or in divided doses.
- The body stores a limited amount of creatine and any excess is excreted. Most people should not exceed 20 grams daily.
- Creatine combined with exercise, especially heavy resistance training, yields the best results.

CHAPTER NINE

What Are the Downsides of Creatine?

SO FAR, YOU have heard about many of the positive aspects of creatine. But creatine, while very safe and usually effective, may also have some downsides. In this chapter, we will examine some of the reported side effects of creatine; how weight gain can be a problem for certain athletes; whether reports of masculinization in women are true; whether there are studies showing long-term safety; if there is evidence of any dangers in using creatine supplements; if there are people who should not use creatine at all; and whether it is ethical to use creatine in sports competitions.

Q: What are some of the common side effects that people using creatine have reported?
A: The most common are cramping, diarrhea and nausea.

Q: What could be the cause of cramping?
A: Cramping is usually related to dehydration and if people drink sufficient liquids and replace electrolytes lost through sweat, most often the cramping disappears.

Q: What are some of the other negative reports that have sur-faced in connection with creatine?
A: People have claimed that it increases the risk of liver and kidney damage, can harm the muscles, and is linked to certain cancers. But there is absolutely no scientific evidence for any of these claims.

Q: Then how do these stories spread?
A: At times, the media may be at fault. Writers can misinterpret a study or get an opinion from someone who is not well informed about the scientific studies and is just passing along bad information. Unfortunately, there are many people who have incorrect beliefs about the supposed dangers of creatine when, in fact, none of these has ever been shown to be true in a properly conducted study. There are also people who have a motivating interest and may intentionally publicize untrue information in order to try to sell their product. That is the case currently with one company selling liquid creatine. They have information on creatine monohydrate powder on their website that is patently false, but many consumers will not know that.

Q: Does this untrue information include reports of so-called side effects, such as cramping, diarrhea and nausea?
A: Yes. Studies have not shown a direct cause-and-effect between creatine use and these side effects. And if we examine people with these complaints, there is usually another reason that can be found, such as dehydration. With regard to gastrointestinal symptoms, a study has found more of a problem in people taking a placebo than in those taking creatine.

Q: Are there any proven side effects that people should be concerned about?
A: The only side effect that has been shown consistently is

weight gain. For a lot of people, especially certain athletes, weight gain is a positive. But for others, it is undesirable.

Q: Which athletes would find weight gain a detriment?
A: As we have already pointed out, long-distance runners, endurance cyclists, and people in sports that require a lot of jumping usually do not want to gain weight. In these sports, extra body mass is a detriment and can harm their performance rather than help it. Also, in sports like swimming and running, where you have to quickly propel yourself, you don't want extra pounds. It's also undesirable for people in sports with weight classes who do not want to be bumped up to the next class, such as boxers, wrestlers, and weight lifters.

Q: Why is it a problem to be pushed into a higher weight class?
A: Athletes try to be as strong and effective as they can pound for pound. For example, take athletes who are competing in a 100-kilogram weight class and are lifting a certain amount of weight. Let's say they use creatine and are bumped slightly over that weight class limit into the next higher class. In this higher class, they will have to compete against others who are much bigger and stronger—they will be at the bottom of that class instead of at the top of their former class. Usually, the athletes who do best are those who are at the upper end of their weight class. If the creatine bumps you up so you are just over your limit, you will have to compete with bigger and stronger people and will have a much harder time succeeding in any competition.

Q: Is dehydration a big problem among creatine users?
A: Dehydration is rarely a problem. Dr. Richard Kreider, one of the foremost creatine researchers, has written that "studies have found that creatine is either without effect or protects against dehydration and cramping."

Q: *How much liquid should people take with their creatine?*
A: Some creatine users say that you should increase your liquid intake when you begin taking creatine supplements, but I haven't seen that in any of the scientific studies. Initially, in the first few days when people load with creatine, they have increased water retention within their muscle cells. That is the opposite of dehydration, so the creatine is definitely not causing dehydration.

During those first few days, there is less urine output because the body is retaining more water. Because of that, it might not be a bad idea to drink a little more water during the loading phase, but it doesn't seem critical. And during the maintenance phase, there is even less to worry about, so extra water should not be necessary. *Adequate* amounts of water, however, are always important.

Q: *Some people have claimed that creatine use increases the risk of injury because larger muscle size can result in muscle pulls and tears, and the fluid retention can cause explosive injuries such as tendon ruptures. Is there any basis for these claims?*
A: All these assertions are without scientific backing. In a 2000 study published in *Medicine and Science in Sports and Exercise,* soccer players were given either creatine or a placebo and during seven weeks of training, the study found that the players using creatine had fewer injuries and as a result, less missed practice than the players who were not taking creatine.

You should also remember that creatine is helpful for people recovering from injuries, so it helps to heal rather than cause injuries.

Q: *Is creatine a risk for growing children under the age of eighteen? Are some reports that it can stunt the growing process actually true?*

A: There have been very few studies on children under eighteen who use creatine, although many do use it. As a result, creatine is generally not recommended for this age group. But I have never seen any scientific evidence that creatine has negative effects on the growth process in children.

Q: *Is there any anecdotal evidence regarding creatine and young children?*
A: Creatine's safety is hinted at by the fact that "Mother Nature" saw fit to put it in human breast milk. Supplemental creatine has been used to successfully treat infants with metabolic disorders without producing any adverse effects, so although there are no definitive studies on safety of creatine in children, the anecdotal evidence has not revealed any dangers.

Q: *What is your recommendation on creatine use in people under the age of eighteen?*
A: At the moment, I don't recommend creatine supplements for adolescents as readily as I would for adults. There haven't been enough studies on children or adolescents for us to feel certain that it is completely safe. And most children under eighteen do not need creatine for any legitimate purpose, with one exception, which is the prevention of traumatic brain injury.

Q: *How can creatine do that?*
A: An animal study found that creatine supplements reduced the severity of traumatic brain damage by up to 50 percent. We can wait for additional studies to be completed, or we can examine the data we have so far and come to a tentative conclusion.

In addition to the study just mentioned, we have other animal studies with similar results and we also have human studies showing the benefit of creatine in certain neurological conditions.

Q: Because of that, do you recommend creatine supplements for certain children?

A: At this point, I am concluding that it is likely that creatine supplementation will reduce the severity of traumatic brain injury in humans. As a consequence, I believe that children participating in high risk sports, such as football, soccer, and ice hockey, may be candidates for creatine supplementation.

However, I do not think that it is easy to decide whether or not these children should use creatine supplementation. At some point, though, we may realize that we are doing more harm than good by not using creatine with children who are at high risk of traumatic brain injury because of the sports they engage in. It is definitely an issue that requires serious thought and discussion.

Q: What if a child under eighteen is already taking creatine? What is your advice?

A: If children are considering the use of creatine, I think before they actually take it, they should make sure they are doing everything they can with their training, that they are very serious about their training and exercise and that they have a good diet and plenty of rest.

In other words, young people should get as much mileage as they can by optimizing their training, diet, rest, and overall lifestyle (see Chapter Eleven). Once they have done that, if they still want to get a little additional competitive edge by using creatine, they should discuss it with their parents and a knowledgeable health care professional. If they are already using it, they should still discuss it and determine if they might perhaps be better off waiting until they are older.

Q: Do you think children need to be monitored if they are using creatine?

A: It's a very good idea. Since they are still growing, they should have periodic examinations to follow their body chemistry and make sure there are no adverse side effects from the creatine supplements. They should also use low doses right from the start, rather than loading, so they don't take a high dose of creatine all at once. And they should use cycling, taking creatine only during the brief period when it's really important for competition, after which they should stop using it.

Q: There have been reports of masculinization in women from using some nutritional supplements, including deeper voices and growth of facial hair. Has creatine been implicated in any of these side effects?
A: These effects are very common with the use of anabolic steroids (see Chapter Ten), but not with creatine. Masculinization in women is a result of elevation of "male" hormones and no such hormonal changes have ever been attributed to creatine, even with studies that specifically looked for them.

You typically see masculinization in women from androgenic hormones, anabolic steroids, or possibly from supplements like androstenedione or DHEA.

Q: What do you see as some of the biggest problems with creatine use?
A: The one issue that seriously concerns me involves the excessive carbohydrates that are often consumed with creatine. A lot of people are using a big load of carbohydrates—90 grams or more—with one dose of creatine, and that is far too much for many individuals.

Q: Why are so many carbohydrates dangerous?
A: With many people, they can have an adverse effect on the physiology. Getting back to masculinization effects in women, one out of ten premenopausal women has a condition called

"androgen dominance." That means they produce too many male hormones and one of the main driving forces behind that is insulin resistance and the associated elevated insulin levels.

Q: *How does this condition develop?*
A: Excess carbohydrates, especially the refined carbohydrates that are used in creatine supplementation, cause a tremendous spike in insulin. One study showed that twenty minutes after taking creatine with 93 grams of carbohydrate, insulin levels were seventeen times higher. Insulin increases the activity of an

George: Creatine Is Sometimes Too Risky

Frail and weak, George came to me as a 77-year-old retired accountant, who looked much older than his years. He suffered from congestive heart failure, walked very slowly, and had difficulty climbing stairs.

Despite his serious health problems, George was determined to improve his condition and was willing to work at it. He especially wanted to have more energy and not to feel sick all the time.

At first, I thought George might benefit from creatine supplementation. But once I had reviewed his blood chemistry results, I found that George had poor kidney function. For that reason, I decided it might not be a good idea for him to use creatine. Even though no scientific proof exists that creatine causes damage to the kidneys, it is filtered through them and would force the kidneys to work harder. I did not want to take any unnecessary chances with George.

Instead, I put George on a weight training program, modified his diet, and recommended other nutritional supplements to support his kidneys. Carefully following this program for several months, George has shown great improvement in strength and energy. In the future, if his kidney function returns to normal, we can consider adding creatine supplements to his regimen.

enzyme in the ovary that converts progesterone to testosterone. So problems with insulin resistance are a major cause of masculinization in women. That's why I have more concern about what the creatine is mixed with rather than with the creatine itself in regard to masculinization of women and side effects in general.

Q: You are saying that the masculinization is actually coming from an excess use of carbohydrates rather than from creatine?
A: That is a definite possibility. If a woman experiences masculinization that is truly, in fact, related to her creatine supplement and not to some other coincidental factor, it is going to be the carbohydrate that is the culprit.

Also, the creatine may not be good quality and people can get various types of symptoms from contaminants in low-grade products. In addition, there are many people who do not use pure creatine monohydrate powder. They purchase products with many different ingredients and then add other compounds on their own, so they may not realize that something else they are taking with the creatine is what is actually causing the unpleasant side effects. It is not the creatine itself.

Q: Are there dangers in using creatine for the long term? There are rumors of liver, kidney, or heart damage, as well as links to certain cancers—do any of them have a foundation in truth?
A: There have been hundreds of studies over many years evaluating athletes and non-athletes who have been using creatine over various periods of time and none has found that creatine has produced any adverse effects. There are more long-term safety data on creatine than on any other ergogenic supplement.

Creatine has been around as a supplement for over thirty years and I think if there were any serious dangers, we would have heard about them by now. But that does not guarantee that adverse side effects may not be found in the future, so to be safe, people should always use creatine according to recommended doses and in the recommended ways.

Q: Can you tell us about some of these studies indicating safety?
A: A 1999 study in *Medicine and Science in Sports and Exercise* showed creatine had no adverse effect on the kidneys in athletes taking it up to five years.

Another study by Kreider entitled "Long term creatine supplementation does not significantly affect clinical markers of health in athletes," presented at an international meeting in 2001, was designed to respond to rumors about creatine's adverse effects. It involved ninety college football players, some of whom received creatine and some of whom did not. The three groups received creatine over different lengths of time: one group for 0-6 months (which included some who got no creatine), another from 7 to 12 months and the last from 12 to 21 months. These athletes were then analyzed for sixty-nine different biochemicals, including measures of liver function, kidney function, red and white blood cells, muscle and liver enzymes, blood lipids and electrolytes. The conclusion was that creatine produced no effect on any of these areas in healthy football players.

Q: What about cancer studies?
A: No scientific connection has ever been found between creatine and cancer in humans. According to Kreider, there are fifteen animal studies showing that creatine has either no effect or a beneficial effect on tumor progression. So these and other studies should put people's minds at rest about any connection between creatine and any form of cancer. Creatine is definitely not a cancer-causing agent.

Q: Are there studies that cover a long period of time?
A: In addition to the studies already mentioned, there are patients with gyrate atrophy who have been taking creatine for close to two decades and who have been carefully monitored for the entire time. They have not shown any adverse effects.

Q: Does all this documentation mean that creatine is completely safe?
A: Even though it appears that way from everything we know, I would not make that statement. Although scientific studies have not yet shown a link between creatine and any adverse health effects, everyone is biochemically different. Due to genetic and various environmental factors, you cannot rule out the possibility of adverse effects in some people.

It is certainly possible that some of the anecdotal reports are true and that creatine can cause minor problems for a small number of individuals. Nothing is one hundred percent safe for everyone. So even if the studies make people feel very comfortable about using it, there is always a small possibility that a person could have an unwanted reaction to creatine.

Q: Have any of your patients reported side effects with creatine?
A: Yes. A small number have reported minor cramps and gastrointestinal distress. There is another condition I have no personal experience with that has been attributed to creatine, and that I think needs to be watched carefully, which is anterior compartment pressure syndrome. The lower leg has muscles, nerves and blood vessels separated into four compartments. Creatine supplementation has been found to increase pressure in the anterior compartment, which is not surprising, since creatine increases muscle mass.

This elevated pressure can rarely produce symptoms of tightness and mild pain in the front of the leg, particularly after activity, and most often in sprinters. So if anyone has these symptoms while using creatine, they should consult a qualified health care professional.

Q: *Have there been any reports of deaths linked to creatine?*
A: No death has ever been linked to creatine. In 1997, there was an inaccurate newspaper report claiming that three college wrestlers had died and that creatine use was implicated, but further investigation found that creatine use was not implicated in any way and that the wrestlers died for different reasons.

Q: *What about other serious health problems?*
A: There have been a small number of cases in which creatine was thought to be linked to kidney failure or kidney damage. But in those cases, once again creatine was not found to be the cause.

Q: *How could such a mistake be made?*
A: One way was that some of the cases were diagnosed using elevated levels of creatinine in the blood as a sign. Creatinine, as you will recall, is a breakdown product of creatine, so when someone is supplementing with creatine, they naturally have a higher level of creatinine. And when the kidneys are not functioning properly, the creatinine is not excreted, so you may get elevated creatinine levels for that reason.

What apparently happened was that someone jumped to the conclusion that there was a direct link between creatine supplementation and kidney problems, whereas the kidney problems were pre-existing and they were the cause of the symptom, rather than the supplemental creatine.

It's interesting to note that weight training can also cause elevated creatinine levels, without the use of any supplemental creatine, and we would not conclude that weight training causes kidney failure. So the source of the problem is not creatine, but something else that is going on in the body, which could be pre-existing kidney problems of which the person is unaware.

Q: Have there been any studies related to this?
A: Regarding creatine safety, Kreider has commented on the fact that some people think it increases renal (kidney) stress or impairs renal function. "These concerns have been primarily fueled by reports of four case studies of possible renal dysfunction in individuals believed to have been taking creatine." He goes on to explain that elevated levels of serum creatinine were used to initially diagnose these cases and that these four individuals either had pre-existing kidney disease, were misdiagnosed or were taking creatine improperly. He concludes that there was no difference in kidney function that could be connected to creatine use.

Q: Could it be dangerous to take too much creatine, especially over a period of many years?
A: Gyrate atrophy patients have taken low doses of creatine for two decades without ill effects. We don't have long-term data on very high doses, but "too much" is too much.

Remember that there is no need to go above the amount of creatine that saturates your muscles, since any excess will be excreted. So it's hard to see that it could have any serious adverse effects, although we really don't know for certain.

To be safe, people should just stick to the short loading phase if they want to load, and then get on a conservative, but effective maintenance dose, which for most people is between 3 and 5 grams a day. It can be higher, up to 10 grams a day, depending on the individual in terms of weight, amount of exercise, age and health.

Q: So your conclusion would be that most people should not take more than 10 grams of creatine a day as a maintenance dose because even if higher amounts may be excreted, we are not certain if they might have bad effects over a period of many years?

A: That would be my conclusion. Be conservative in your use of creatine and follow the established guidelines, and you should not have any problems.

Q: *Are there people who should not take creatine at all or who need to be carefully monitored if they use it?*

A: Yes. Although they are in the minority, it is very important to know if you are one of them. People who have kidney or liver conditions should probably not use creatine, or at least they should get their physician's approval and be monitored if they use it. Creatine use does not cause kidney or liver problems. However, if there is a pre-existing dysfunction in either of these organs, creatine may be too much of a burden. People who take any medication that has an effect on the liver or kidneys should also be monitored by physicians. And pregnant women or women who want to become pregnant should not use creatine because there have been no studies that prove its safety. The same is true for young children. There are some studies involving teenagers, but as we have already said, they should only use creatine with caution and medical supervision.

If creatine is used in any of these questionable situations, it is wise to use only a maintenance dose, which is not drastically different from the amount of creatine you get from our diet. Results may take longer than with loading creatine, but it is a safer way to go.

There are times when people have health conditions and are not aware of it, and that's why it is always a good idea to have a thorough medical examination prior to taking any supplement, even creatine, which is safer than most.

Q: What about ethics? Is it ethical to get a boost from using creatine for sports competitions? Does it give people who use it an unfair advantage over those who do not?

A: That is a question each person has to answer individually. Some of the dangerous supplements, such as steroids, have been banned by most sports organizations, but creatine falls into a gray area.

Q: What do you mean by a "gray area"?

A: There is not always a black and white division between "natural" and "drug." Creatine is somewhere in between the two. Creatine is a naturally occurring compound, but when it is used in supplemental form, it produces an effect that you would never achieve without using it as a supplement, since you are going beyond the creatine you would normally get in your diet. It has been compared to taking vitamins in pill form rather than getting them just from food. Creatine supplementation has also been likened to carbohydrate loading.

I think that all things being equal, athletes who are supplementing with creatine are going to have an edge over their competitors, and the athletes who do not take creatine supplements are going to be at a disadvantage in the sports where creatine has a beneficial effect.

But is it ethical? I can't answer that question for others. For myself, I believe that while I am not one hundred percent in favor of using any performance-enhancing substance, I lean towards using creatine because of its effectiveness and apparent safety.

Q: If you had identical twins and one was using creatine supplements and the other was not, the one taking creatine would perform better in weight lifting, for example?

A: That would almost certainly be the case.

Q: *But not everyone who takes creatine is going to be outstanding or a winner in his or her sport?*
A: No. The creatine should help, but it will not mean the difference between being a mediocre athlete and suddenly becoming a champion. Creatine provides a boost, but it doesn't perform miracles.

Q: *Do you think things would be better if supplements like creatine did not exist and sports competitions could be more "natural?"*
A: Possibly. But for the many health benefits it provides, I am glad we have creatine supplements. In today's complicated world, if you wanted to make competitions equal, you would have to create divisions for people who use creatine and those who do not, people who use protein supplements and those who do not, and so on.

In short, it would not be possible to make everything equal. So we have to face the fact that we do not enter sports competitions on a level playing field. It is completely understandable that people try to get an edge—it's just human nature. If they try to get that edge by using creatine, it doesn't seem like such a terrible thing to do. We work out, practice, try to eat a good diet, get enough rest, and so on. Adding a little supplemental creatine from time to time is one way of getting a boost and maximizing your potential without any real harm. So yes, overall I'm in favor of it.

Points to Remember

- The most commonly reported side effects from people taking creatine are cramping, diarrhea, and nausea, but none of these has been scientifically linked to creatine use.

- Other reports, including those involving kidney, liver and heart problems, and links to cancer, are also completely without scientific support.
- Weight gain is the only documented unwanted side effect from creatine use, since it can be a detriment to certain athletes, including long-distance runners, swimmers, cyclists, and those who do not want to move into a higher weight class in such sports as weight lifting, boxing, and wrestling.
- Contrary to rumor, creatine does not cause dehydration. But it needs to be accompanied by sufficient liquid intake.
- Creatine is not generally recommended for children under the age of eighteen. If they use it, medical supervision and parental consent are strongly advised.
- Taking high doses of carbohydrates with creatine has the potential to cause serious problems with insulin levels and consequent unwanted side effects in certain individuals.
- No deaths have ever been linked to creatine use.
- Individuals have to decide whether using creatine to get a competitive edge is ethical.

CHAPTER TEN

Other Muscle-Building Supplements

YOU HAVE SEEN that creatine appears to be very safe and effective in terms of building muscle and strength. But creatine is only one of many such substances. In this chapter, you will learn about some of the other supplements that people use to build muscle and strength. You will discover if they are as effective or even better than creatine; whether some of them work best when combined with creatine or other substances; and whether some of the available supplements are dangerous and should be avoided. We will also look at which supplements have been banned by sports organizations and why.

Q: In addition to creatine, what are some of the more popular muscle-building supplements that athletes use?
A: There are quite a few, including protein supplements; supplements that are referred to as "weight-gainers" that are usually a combination of a lot of protein and carbohydrates with high overall calories; HMB, which is beta-hydroxy-beta-methylbutyrate; androstenedione (also called "andro") and related hor-

mones; DHEA, which stands for dehydroepiandrosterone; vanadyl sulfate; tribulus terrestris; glutamine; chromium; pyruvate; and magnesium. Of course, there are others as well, but these are some of the ones most commonly used.

Q: Which are the most dangerous and/or banned?
A: Anabolic steroids appear to be the most dangerous muscle-building substances. They are synthetic androgenic compounds and are banned in many different sports.

Q: Exactly what are they and how do they work?
A: Anabolic steroids are very similar to the body's own testosterone, or male hormones, but they are distinctly different. Because of that difference, there is a lot of toxicity associated with their use. The body has complex regulatory mechanisms to keep hormones in relative balance. When you take synthetic compounds like anabolic steroids, that have a different chemical structure, the body doesn't have the control to regulate their activity. In other words, the body can't detoxify them efficiently and so much greater adverse side effects can occur. They are a lot more dangerous than natural testosterone.

Q: What organizations have banned anabolic steroids?
A: They are banned by many organizations, including the International Olympic Committee, the NCAA, pro football, and many other professional sports. Major league baseball has recently decided to ban them, as well.

Q: Can you give us more details about anabolic steroids?
A: Anabolic steroids are synthetic androgenic (or male) hormones. Testosterone is the main male hormone and is found in both men and women, but in much higher levels in men. The production of testosterone is greatly increased during puberty

and gives rise to secondary sexual characteristics in men. These include the development of muscle mass, deepening of the voice, and growth of facial hair. Testosterone also has other beneficial influences in men and women, contributing to bone density, libido, and a positive mood.

Q: *Are there any beneficial uses for anabolic steroids?*
A: Yes. They have been used in medicine for certain conditions, often with good results. For example, people with wasting conditions like HIV infections, can benefit from a course of anabolic steroids to help them gain muscle mass. They have also been used for certain types of breast cancer, certain rare forms of anemia, and other conditions.

Years ago, when the general public learned that anabolic steroids help to build muscle mass and increase strength, many power athletes, such as weight lifters, football players, and bodybuilders, in particular, began to obtain and use them.

Q: *Why are they dangerous and what are some of the unwanted side effects of anabolic steroids?*
A: There are many. First of all, you're increasing the body's androgen levels above normal and secondly, the steroids are not natural compounds, the body doesn't have appropriate means to detoxify them. That's why athletes typically cycle steroids on and off, so they can give their bodies a little break from some of the negative side effects.

The body also converts anabolic steroids into other hormones that can give rise to certain unwanted side effects. For example, in men, the size of breasts can increase, while in women, steroids can reduce the size of the breasts and cause growth of facial hair, deepening of the voice, and acne. These are the masculinization effects we mentioned before.

Q: *What are some of the other possible side effects of anabolic steroids?*

A: They include sterility, shrinking of the testicles, impotence, loss of hair, sleep disturbances, high cholesterol levels, liver damage, increased cancer growth, and a tendency to act violently, which is commonly referred to as "roid rage."

Anabolic steroids are so widely banned because they have so many negative, unhealthy side effects, and because they give athletes who take them a very unfair advantage over those who do not. We should also point out that anabolic steroids are illegal in the United States unless they are obtained by prescription for a legitimate health reason.

Q: *Despite all these dangers, are anabolic steroids still widely used?*

A: Yes. Some recent studies indicate that as many as two million people in this country, including half a million adolescents, have used anabolic steroids at some time. And their use is on the rise. One 2001 survey found that the use of steroids and other similar drugs was up 25 percent in just one year (1999–2000). People have many different motivations for using them. According to surveys, they include wanting to put on more muscle, to look better, and to compete more effectively in their sports.

One of the most disturbing recent findings is that illegal anabolic steroids are being used by boys as young as ten years old in order to improve their physical appearance. In fact, many high school boys have been arrested for selling steroids, and it is a situation that appears to be getting worse. So even though the serious dangers of steroid use are widely known, young boys who want to look better and put on muscle quickly ignore all the warnings. It's a very bad situation.

Q: What is the cause of "roid rage?"
A: I think that most of the time when people are using steroids, they are prone to taking an excessive dose. They think that if a little is good, then more will be better. So they believe that if they use a lot, they will build bigger muscles and do it more quickly. But these high levels in the body can cause extreme changes in the personality, including mood swings, sudden outbursts of anger, and unprovoked physical violence. Steroid use has even been implicated in suicides and murder, which can occur when people are unable to control their violent or extreme impulses. Because of these and other negative consequences, anabolic steroids are not something that people should be using in any amount.

Q: After anabolic steroids, what are some other dangerous muscle-building compounds?
A: I think the second most dangerous compounds are related to anabolic steroids, namely other hormones such as androstenedione and its derivatives, followed by DHEA.

Q: If they are dangerous, why are they used so often?
A: Because people believe that these supplements are going to help them build muscle and improve performance. But the fact is that even if some of them do build muscle and improve performance, others do not. And all of them have potentially very serious side effects that people should avoid. No one should use any of these substances for muscle building or to improve sports performance.

Q: Why don't people heed that advice?
A: It has to do with the psychological makeup of certain people. Competitors often want to win at any cost. They want to get bigger and build more muscle, and they refuse to believe any of the

negative reports they may hear. It's the "it can't happen to me" type of thinking. They focus totally on the potential benefits and ignore the negative side effects, even when the negatives become very evident to everyone else.

In other cases, people are simply not well informed. They use various substances because their friends are using them and getting good results, but they have little or no information on what they are ingesting and what it can do to their bodies and they make no effort to find out.

So people have different attitudes towards supplements. Some people are very cautious, investigate everything thoroughly, take very few supplements, and use only what they are convinced is safe. Others will take anything without even giving it a second thought, as long as they see some potential benefit in using it.

Q: Androstenedione has been readily available for many years and used by many athletes, including Mark McGwire. How similar is it to a steroid?
A: Androstenedione is similar to a steroid. Steroid molecules are a class of compounds that have a certain chemical structure. Vitamin D, cholesterol, and many hormones belong to the same class. So steroids include not only anabolic steroids, but testosterone, mineralcorticoids, estrogen, progesterone, DHEA and glucocorticoids, the stress hormones in the adrenal glands.

Androstenedione is one of the steroid hormones that is produced by the adrenal glands. It is an androgenic hormone and has some influence on male secondary sexual characteristics. So in that way, it is similar to anabolic steroids. I don't think andro is as dangerous as anabolic steroids, but it is also not as effective in building muscle and strength. Andro is available in health food stores and is heavily marketed to bodybuilders.

Q: Do you think it is safe to use andro?
A: I don't. The average consumer reads the promotional literature and is probably taken in. But if you look at the research on andro, you will find that most of the claims are without merit. In my opinion, it's pretty much a waste of money, and it could have dangerous side effects, as well.

Q: Can you present some information on one of the andro studies you're referring to?
A: A 1999 study that appeared in *The Journal of the American Medical Association* (*JAMA*) concluded that andro does not increase serum testosterone concentrations or enhance skeletal muscle adaptations to resistance training in normal young men and "may result in adverse health conditions."

The premise behind andro is that it is converted to testosterone in the body, so the body will then produce higher testosterone levels, which will increase muscle mass and strength. It sounds logical, but in reality, it doesn't work.

There are other studies as well showing that people undergoing resistance training with andro and without andro have the same results in terms of strength and body composition. They all conclude that andro does not appear to alter body composition.

Q: Does that mean that the people who have taken andro and think it has helped build muscle are wrong?
A: It's hard to say. It may work in some people, but I don't think it works for most. Every published study I have examined has found andro to be without merit in terms of increasing strength or muscle.

Q: You also mentioned DHEA in the same group?
A: Yes. DHEA is a hormone made by the adrenal glands and is widely used as a nutritional supplement. There is evidence that

it may be converted to testosterone in the body, but there is no scientific evidence that it helps to build muscle or increase physical strength in young men. There is one study that found that older men got stronger by using DHEA. Like anabolic steroids and andro, it has the potential for serious side effects, including masculinization in women, insomnia, headaches, irritability and even liver damage. However, it is much safer than anabolic steroids and also safer than andro.

For men to take DHEA in the hope that their bodies will convert it to testosterone and build more muscle is a leap of faith. DHEA may convert to testosterone, but like androstenedione, in male bodies it appears to raise estrogen levels to an even greater extent. Inflammation and excess body fat accelerate the conversion to estrogen. This is not a recipe for strength and muscle building, although each individual will respond in a unique way. Women, on the other hand, do usually experience an increase in testosterone levels from taking DHEA.

Q: What are your recommendations regarding andro and DHEA as muscle-building supplements?
A: I recommend that no one consider taking these hormones without first having some laboratory testing done. I regularly test these hormones in my patients, mainly with salivary analysis. The hormones show up in their active form in the saliva, which is easy to collect. If someone has a low DHEA level, it can be a good idea to use DHEA supplements just to raise it to the normal level. You can test for levels of testosterone, estrogen, progesterone, and androstenedione as well.

Sometimes I find individuals who have elevated levels of DHEA or andro. To further increase levels, as might be done through "blind" supplementing, is dangerous. Once you are taking supplements to raise your levels to normal, you will be retested. From subsequent tests, you can see how much is being con-

Ed: Speeding Recovery from Injury

Ed was a 39-year-old bank manager and dedicated racquetball player. He came to me seeking relief from lower back pain. After working with him for a while, Ed came in one day on crutches. He explained that he had been running across a street when he fell and felt as if his calf had been hit with a golf ball. He consulted an orthopedic surgeon and discovered that he had a ruptured Achilles' tendon. He underwent surgery and the surgeon said he would be on crutches for about three months. Naturally, Ed was very unhappy about this turn of events and asked me if there was anything we could do to hasten his recovery.

I developed a program for Ed, including proteolytic enzymes, bioflavonoids, glucosamine sulfate, and other supplements that would help his injury to heal more quickly and completely. Because of research findings that creatine can aid with rehabilitation after injury, I suggested that Ed take a powder containing creatine monohydrate, glutamine, dextrose, and maltodextrin.

After about a month, Ed was able to walk without crutches. He then began a program of rehabilitation exercise and made rapid progress. After another two and a half months, Ed was playing racquetball again.

Ed continues to cycle creatine on and off because it makes him feel stronger, and he also feels that his racquetball game has benefited from the supplement, giving him increased power and speed. Based on creatine studies, it is also likely that creatine can help Ed to avoid other injuries in the future.

verted to testosterone or to estrogen and how your individual body is reacting to the supplements.

The action of hormones in the body is very complex and unique to each individual, so people should not take these substances as though they are candy. It's playing with fire because they can cause some very serious side effects.

Q: You mentioned testosterone. What about using supplemental testosterone in order to improve sports performance?
A: As with the other hormones, you would only want to use supplemental testosterone under medical supervision in the event that your body's natural levels are depleted. But rather than taking additional testosterone, people usually do better with an approach that increases the body's own release of testosterone. That is what should be tried first. If boosting the body's own production doesn't work, then testosterone replacement may be beneficial.

Q: Are there any studies on supplementary testosterone?
A: Yes. A 1996 study divided the subjects into four groups: a placebo group with no exercise, a placebo group with exercise, a testosterone group with no exercise and a testosterone group with exercise. The researchers found that taking testosterone produced an increase in muscle mass and strength, but when it was combined with exercise, the results were much better.

So the testosterone increased fat-free mass, muscle size and strength. It does work. But the potential side effects, especially in large doses and/or over a long period of time, can be very serious.

Q: Athletes are also using human growth hormone to improve their performance. Is it safe?
A: The use of human growth hormone is very controversial. It has both benefits and dangers and is still being widely studied. Bodybuilders and weight lifters, among others, sometimes take it in very large amounts, but there are few studies to show whether or not it works and whether or not it is safe.

A recent study published in 2002 in *JAMA* concluded that human growth hormone can benefit older people by helping to build body mass and decrease body fat, even though they did not exercise or change their diets. The subjects, ranging in age from their sixties to eighties, also developed unwanted side effects, including diabetes, aching joints, and swollen tissues. This is an indication that human growth hormone may have adverse long-term effects, but that is not certain, since this study covered only a six-month period.

Growth hormone can also foster tumor growth and contribute to carpal tunnel syndrome. In animals, growth hormone injections seem to improve quality of life but also shorten life span. So from what we know at this time, it's a double-edged sword, and I think most people would want to stay away from it.

Q: What about the use of glutamine supplements?
A: There is a good rationale for using glutamine supplements. Glutamine is the most abundant amino acid in muscle, and when the body is under stress and needs glutamine, it goes to the muscle for it, causing tissue breakdown. That results in metabolic stress to the body, so there is a good reason to supplement with glutamine. So far, studies have not shown any significant effect on muscle building or performance, but I do recommend that people consider taking some supplemental glutamine.

Studies with cancer and AIDS patients who were wasting (losing excessive body weight) found that a combination of glutamine, arginine, and HMB produced gains in body weight and muscle mass.

Q: Aside from its possible effect on muscle building, does glutamine have other benefits?
A: Quite a few. It's an important fuel source for lymphocytes, the white blood cells that protect us against viruses and cancer cells. It's also the main fuel source for the cells that line the small intestine, and those cells are very important to the health of the body because they have the important dual function of absorb-

ing nutrients and keeping toxins from the intestinal tract out of the bloodstream. Glutamine also plays an important role in the body's acid-base balance.

So even though glutamine hasn't been shown to produce measurable effects so far on muscle growth and strength, further studies might show otherwise in the future. In the meantime, I recommend glutamine for its health benefits.

Q: Glutamine is only one of many amino acids. How do people know which ones they might need?
A: If you want to get a good idea of which amino acids might benefit you, I recommend doing an amino acid analysis. That can be performed with urine or blood specimens or both. This analysis will determine which amino acids may be lacking in your body and which ones you may want to take in the form of supplements.

The analysis will also let you see if you are getting adequate dietary protein or if you might be getting too much protein. Too much protein is a common finding with bodybuilders. It also gives a lot of evidence regarding the need for various vitamins and minerals and indicators regarding the body's ability to digest and absorb foods, so it can be very useful for people who want to know exactly what nutrients they need.

Amino acid supplements, however, can be used for purposes other than correcting a deficiency. When it comes to strength and muscle building, it is interesting to note that supplementation of two of the amino acids that make up creatine, arginine and glycine, has been demonstrated to increase creatine levels. Amino acids can be taken for therapeutic or pharmacologic actions.

Q: Are there any studies that demonstrate the effect of amino acids on building strength?

A: In a 1989 double-blind placebo-controlled study, twenty-two men took either an arginine and orthinine supplement, or a placebo and then underwent a five-week strength training program. The subjects taking the arginine-orthinine combination experienced greater gains in strength and lean body mass.

In another double-blind cross-over study, an evaluation was made of the immediate effects on exercise of an amino acid mixture versus a sugar placebo. The amino acid mixture consisted of glycine, arginine and the leucine metabolite, alpha-ketoisocaproic acid. It was found that the amino acid mixture increased strength and overall muscle performance and delayed fatigue.

Q: What can you tell us about chromium supplements and muscle building?
A: In most studies, chromium has been found to produce no effect on muscle building. One 1998 study, for example, which appeared in *Medicine and Science in Sports and Exercise* with Walker as the lead author, found that chromium picolinate produced no effect on body composition or performance variables, which were upper body endurance and bench press power.

The rationale behind chromium supplements is that it will improve the way insulin works in the body and will also increase muscle mass and strength. But so far, there is no scientific evidence that shows a favorable effect.

Q: Many athletes also use pyruvate. Is there any positive evidence on this supplement?
A: Pyruvate has not been extensively studied and at this time, cannot be recommended for muscle building. In one study, it was combined with creatine and the group that used both creatine and pyruvate, as well as the group using only creatine, both had beneficial changes in muscle mass and strength, but there were no changes in the group that used only pyruvate.

Q: So we can assume that it was the creatine that had the beneficial effect?
A: I think so. You have to remember that no nutritional supplement has the research backing that creatine does and no nutritional supplement can compare with creatine in terms of building muscle mass and strength.

Q: Whey protein is another supplement popular with athletes. Does it work?
A: I think there is some value to whey protein. One of the factors that may influence whether a person responds to whey protein is how much protein they are getting from their diet already. There definitely are people who do not eat enough protein. And if, on the other hand, you eat too much protein, there can also be negative side effects. So if you use whey protein supplements, you have to be careful about how much you use. Many bodybuilders and strength athletes consume too much protein.

Q: How much protein should people have?
A: One widely accepted recommendation is 1.3 to 1.8 grams of protein per kilogram of body weight. But each person's protein needs are individual, and these needs can also change, depending on conditions such as how much activity the person gets or the amount of stress that is in their lives at any given time.

Q: Are there studies showing whey protein's beneficial effects for athletes?
A: Yes. One appeared in 2001 in the *International Journal of Sports Nutrition and Exercise Metabolism,* with Burk as the lead author. In this study, thirty-six males divided into three groups went through six weeks of resistance training. The first group received a placebo, the second whey protein, and the third whey protein and creatine.

The group receiving creatine and whey protein showed the best results. The group on whey protein alone did have an increase in knee extension, peak torque, and in lean tissue mass greater than the placebo group.

Q: In general, does the need for supplemental protein increase with age?
A: There is some evidence that it does. One 2001 study in the *Journal of Gerontology* concluded that "the recommended dietary allowance for protein may not be adequate for older people to maintain skeletal muscle."

Q: What is in whey protein and is it the best form of protein for building muscle?
A: Whey protein is comprised of 25 percent branched chain amino acids, has all the essential amino acids in high levels, and it also has high levels of glutamic acid, which is readily converted to glutamine. It has relatively high levels of tryptophan, which may contribute to better mood. It is also a source of sulfur, which is critical for connective tissue health. Whey protein is a rich source of antibodies and other immune-boosting compounds.

There is also one study indicating that casein (a protein produced when milk curdles) can produce better results in terms of building muscle mass and strength. So at this time, we really can't say that whey protein is absolutely the best or only form of protein that should be used as a muscle-building supplement, although it is my first choice.

Q: HMB (beta-hydroxy-beta-methylbutyrate) is another popular supplement. Do you think it works?
A: HMB is a metabolite of the branched-chain amino acid, leucine. The studies on HMB are mixed, with some showing benefits and others showing no effect. Overall, I would say that it is worth con-

sidering only if you are very serious about muscle building, because it is quite expensive. Also, in order to take it at the dosages used in the studies, you would have to take twelve capsules a day.

In the studies where it worked, HMB increased muscle mass and also decreased body fat. In one study, it appeared to reduce damage to muscles from exercise, and in another, it produced decreases in total cholesterol, LDL cholesterol and blood pressure. In another study where HMB was combined with creatine, the supplements together produced benefits in terms of increased fat-free mass and strength, which were greater than when either substance was used alone.

So overall, I am in favor of HMB. It has good safety data although studies do not go back as far as those with creatine. So if you want to pay the money and experiment to find out if HMB does something for you, I think that's fine.

Q: *What is your opinion of* Tribulus terrestris?
A: This is an herbal supplement that has been widely used, especially in Europe, but not studied too much. I've seen one study, which appeared in the *International Journal of Sports Nutrition and Exercise Metabolism* in 2000, where tribulus produced no effect. The study found that tribulus supplements did not enhance body composition or exercise performance in resistance trained males. Until there is some evidence that it works, I cannot recommend it.

Q: *Some experts say that magnesium is an important supplement for athletes. Is that true?*
A: Magnesium is a mineral that is widely deficient in the typical American diet. It is a coenzyme for about 80 percent of the enzymes in the body. A coenzyme is a substance that is required for the enzyme to do its job. So when people are deficient in magnesium, there can be many negative effects.

For that reason alone, I think that magnesium supplements could make a difference in sports performance, especially for those who are lacking the required amounts from their diets.

Q: Are there any studies showing the effectiveness of magnesium supplements on exercise?
A: Yes. A 2001 study in the *Canadian Journal of Applied Physiology* found that "magnesium and zinc play significant roles in promoting strength."

In a 1992 double-blind placebo controlled trial, with Brilla as the lead researcher, twenty-six subjects underwent a seven-week resistance training program. The group receiving a magnesium supplement experienced greater gains in strength.

Another study of alcoholics who were deficient in magnesium found that muscle strength increased significantly when they were given magnesium supplements.

Q: How much magnesium should people take?
A: I recommend that people take a potent multivitamin and mineral supplement that contains magnesium, but that will not be sufficient because you can't fit enough magnesium into one pill. So for most people, I recommend a separate magnesium supplement with about 300–500 milligrams of elemental magnesium, which is a pretty good dose. If you want to get the benefits, you need at least a few hundred milligrams a day. It is important to take a form that is well absorbed and will not cause diarrhea in large doses. One such form is magnesium glycinate. Magnesium aspartate is another good form for athletes.

Q: Is vanadyl sulfate a good supplement for muscle building?
A: Vanadyl sulfate is a form of the mineral vanadium, which some people believe is effective in building muscle and increasing energy. But there is very little documentation on this supple-

ment. One study in a 1996 issue of the *International Journal of Sports and Nutrition* found that vanadyl sulfate was not effective in changing body composition in weight training athletes. So I would not recommend it at this time.

Q: *Are there any other supplements that we should mention?*
A: Colostrum, which is the first milk that a mammal produces when nursing, has been tested for its effects on body composition and exercise performance in men and women. One study published in 2001 in *Nutrition* found that the group that was supplemented with colostrum "experienced a significant increase in bone-free lean body mass." The researchers went on to say that in combination with exercise training over an eight-week period, bovine colostrum "may increase bone-free lean body mass in active men and women."

Colostrum is very high in antibodies and growth factors and has been used by bodybuilders. It appears to be beneficial for the immune system and according to this study, it may also have a positive effect on muscle mass.

Another substance that could be useful is ginseng. A 2000 review of supplements and herbs in the *American Journal of Clinical Nutrition,* by Luke Bucci, Ph.D., found that a number of different supplements and herbs can be useful for athletes. While many of them appeared to have little or no value, he found that Asian ginseng caused "improvements in exercise perform-ance" under certain conditions. These conditions included the use of standardized root extracts, use for more than eight weeks, a daily dose of more than 1 gram of dried root or the equivalent, and a large number of subjects and older subjects. Under these conditions, one of the improvements noted was muscular strength.

My conclusion from what I've seen on ginseng is that athletes over the age of forty might benefit from using very high-quality ginseng. You would really have to consult a knowledgeable nutritionist or herbalist to be certain you are getting the best quality.

Q: Athletes are using a lot of supplements, including some that are illegal, to boost performance. Some of these appear to work and others don't. Do many sports organizations test for these substances?

A: There isn't too much testing in sports until you get to the highest levels, such as the Olympics or major league baseball or pro football, for example. And even then, they usually only test randomly and are unable to test for many of the substances that are being used, since effective tests have not yet been developed. I think that the use of supplements is very widespread, is often unwise, and can frequently have unwanted or dangerous side effects. People really have to respect their bodies, take only what they find out they need and only what they can use safely.

Points to Remember

- In addition to creatine, many other supplements are used by those who want to build muscle.
- Some of these supplements appear to be effective, but many do not. Unlike creatine, most of them have not been well studied.
- More popular supplements include whey protein, HMB, androstenedione, DHEA, vanadyl sulfate, *Tribulus terrestris,* glutamine, chromium, pyruvate, magnesium, and anabolic steroids, which are illegal and very dangerous.
- Despite well-documented dangers, the use of anabolic steroids is rapidly increasing, with boys as young as ten using them to bulk up and improve their looks.
- Androstenedione or "andro," legal but similar to anabolic steroids, may not be quite as dangerous, but is also not very effective and not recommended.

144 • THE ULTIMATE CREATINE HANDBOOK

- Athletes use supplements of testosterone and human growth hormone to improve performance, but both can have very serious side effects and are not recommended.
- Certain supplements appear to be of special benefit to older adults in terms of improving muscle mass and strength.
- There is very little testing in organized sports for most of these supplements. However, anabolic steroids are widely banned and tested for, although their rate of use appears to be rapidly growing.
- It is very important to be knowledgeable about supplements and to take only those you really need and know are safe and effective.

CHAPTER ELEVEN

Creatine and Anti-Aging

TODAY, ANTI-AGING IS one of the most important areas in health and nutrition. We now realize that while the breakdown of the body is inevitable, there are things we can do to slow the aging process, and both men and women are doing everything they can to remain as young as possible for as long as possible. When it comes to anti-aging, most of us think of plastic surgery, Botox, special diets, and exercise. Because of its unique properties, creatine can be a significant part of an effective anti-aging program. In this chapter, we will look at what causes the signs of aging, how we can hold back the body's decline, and where creatine fits in.

Q: Why are men and women so concerned about staying young?
A: One reason is because our society emphasizes looking young and fit and those ideas are ingrained in us from a young age. Then when people reach middle age, they begin to witness a decline in their parents and others. They see a decrease in qual-

ity of life, long periods of illness, and loss of mental faculties. These observations motivate them to find ways to remain vibrant and active as long as they can.

Q: Can you give us some details about the aging process itself? What causes the symptoms we experience as we grow older?
A: First let's look at the difference between biological and chronological age. Looking at your driver's license, you see your chronological age, which is how many revolutions you've done around the sun. But your biological age, which can be quite different, is the age of the tissues in your body and your level of functioning.

We all know people who look much younger or much older than their chronological age. That's because biological age differs from person to person. So biological aging, which is aging of the physical body, is associated with damage to the tissues of the body. And that occurs primarily through the process of oxidative stress or the action of free radicals.

Q: What are free radicals?
A: They are highly reactive molecules with an unpaired electron. Free radicals steal electrons from other molecules in order to make themselves stable. But in the process of doing that, they create another free radical, and in this way, they perpetuate a chain of electron stripping. That continues until all the free radicals are neutralized by compounds that can donate electrons without becoming free radicals themselves.

The compounds that neutralize free radicals and stop their damage to the body are called antioxidants.

Q: How do free radicals damage the body's tissues?
A: They alter and damage the tissues, and that also impairs the body's functions. We all have free radicals coursing through our

bodies all the time—there is no way to get away from them. Free radicals are a byproduct of energy production.

However, increased free radical production is seen in inflammation, toxicity, and states of insulin resistance. But a healthy body has the means to keep free radicals in check and reduce the damage they cause.

If you look at free radical activity in different species, you can see the damage. The fruit fly, for example, experiences a tremendous amount of free radical activity in its body, and that could have a lot to do with its very short lifespan.

Q: What specific signs of aging does free radical damage cause?
A: It causes tissue damage and loss of function, which can be seen from the subcellular level all the way up to the level of the whole person, in such things as the ability to get around, to stand up and get out of a chair, to walk a flight of stairs, to engage in cognitive functions, to remember, or to reason. Skin wrinkling, heart disease, arthritis, cancer, and Alzheimer's disease are a few of the conditions linked to free-radical damage.

Q: Are there certain significant markers for aging?
A: Yes, there are. One that is commonly used is grip strength. Using an instrument called a hand dynamometer, an individual's grip strength can be measured and compared with chronological age. So a person who is thirty years old may have the strength of a fifty-year-old, and a fifty-year-old may have the strength of a thirty-year-old.

Weaker grip strength in middle age correlates with greater disability in later life and with decreased life span. Incidentally, creatine supplementation has been found to increase grip strength.

Another marker is muscle mass. Aging is associated with a decline in muscle. The book *Biomarkers,* by Evans and

Rosenberg, lists some of the top markers that are associated with the aging process.

Q: *How does creatine fit in on this list?*
A: In the book, the number-one biomarker is muscle mass, followed by strength. Since creatine has been shown to be the best supplement for improving both muscle mass and strength, we could easily call it the ultimate anti-aging nutrient.

Q: *What other anti-aging benefits does creatine appear to have?*
A: Creatine has been found to improve resting metabolic rate, which is the number-three biomarker, according to Evans and Rosenberg. Creatine also apparently improves mitochondrial function (subcellular organelles involved in energy production). Mitochondrial damage has been linked to many age-associated diseases, including cancer, heart disease, Alzheimer's disease, and neural degeneration.

A 2001 study in *Metabolism* entitled "Comparison of creatine ingestion and resistance training on energy expenditure and limb blood flow," divided subjects into three groups. One group received only creatine. The other two groups underwent a resistance training program and took either creatine or a placebo. One of the interesting results of this study was that the group that exercised and took creatine had a significant increase (30 and 38 percent, respectively) in calf and forearm blood flow, whereas the other two groups did not.

Increased blood flow is important for health in general, and in particular, for intermittent claudication, which is a disease of the arteries in the legs that impairs one's ability to walk any distance without disabling pain. Once again, weight training and creatine are found to be a dynamic duo!

Studies have also shown that creatine acts as an antioxidant and is often helpful when used with the elderly.

Q: Can you cite a study that demonstrates this?
A: A 2001 study published in *Medicine and Science in Sports and Exercise* looked at thirty men with an average age of 70.4 years. The subjects were divided into two groups: one was given creatine and the other a placebo. Then both groups were weight trained. At the end of the study period, the group given creatine had a greater increase in fat-free mass, knee extension strength and endurance, leg press endurance and overall power. The conclusion: "Creatine supplementation, when combined with resistance training, increases lean tissue mass and improves leg strength, endurance, and average power in men with a mean age of 70 years."

Other studies with creatine and older subjects have also found benefits in terms of building muscle strength and helping people to perform tasks of everyday life with greater ease. One of these studies concluded, "Creatine supplementation may be a useful therapeutic strategy for older adults to attenuate loss in muscle strength and performance of functional living tasks."

Q: What effects does creatine have on the cells that could reverse signs of aging?
A: One of the things creatine does is increase intracellular water, which is the amount of body water located within the cells. Intracellular water tends to decrease with age. As we grow older, there is a shift of water from inside to outside the cells, due to a weakening of the cell membranes or to a decline in cellular energy levels, resulting in failure of "pumps" on the membrane. Creatine both increases cellular energy and stabilizes cellular membranes. After only a few days of using creatine, intracellular water increases. I know this because it is something I routinely measure with my patients.

Q: You said that creatine acts like an antioxidant. Can you explain more about that?
A: A 2002 study by Lawler and associates, entitled "Direct antioxidant properties of creatine," found that creatine was a potent antioxidant in protecting against certain highly reactive free radicals. So by helping to neutralize free radicals, creatine can have a beneficial effect on the aging process.

Q: You mentioned that a condition called insulin resistance can be helped by creatine. Does insulin resistance also cause age-related problems?
A: Yes, very definitely. When the body is working properly, the pancreas secretes insulin, a hormone that helps transport nutrients from the blood into the cells. Glucose is the most important of these. When the cells don't respond efficiently to insulin signals to transport glucose, the pancreas responds by overcompensating. In other words, it goes into overdrive and begins to turn out more insulin in order to do its job. Eventually, if this continues, people will develop high blood insulin levels, which can have serious effects on health.

Q: What are some of the things that can happen if this occurs?
A: You can develop very high cholesterol and triglyceride levels, diabetes, obesity, cardiovascular disease, hypertension, certain cancers, Alzheimer's disease, fatigue, inflammation, osteoporosis, depression, and fibromyalgia, among others. So insulin resistance definitely accelerates the aging process.

An example that confirms this is a 2001 study by Facchini published in *The Journal of the American Medical Association*, that looked at the connection between insulin resistance and the development of age-associated diseases. The study involved 208 healthy men who were evaluated for their insulin sensitivity and then followed for an average of six years. After the study period, one out of every three men in the study who had insulin resistance had developed high blood pressure, type 2 diabetes, cancer, heart disease, or stroke. And all of the men who had good insulin metabolism remained healthy.

Q: *About what percentage of the population has insulin resistance problems?*
A: It has been estimated at about 25 percent, and that is a conservative estimate.

Q: *What about blood sugar tolerance?*
A: That is related to insulin resistance. Sugar and insulin are connected. Initially, when there are problems with insulin, blood sugar may remain in the normal range, but there are other negative consequences, as we just mentioned. If the cells continue to further lose their sensitivity, the pancreas cannot meet the demands for transporting sugar into the blood and blood sugar rises. When it reaches a certain level, diabetes develops. Creatine has an impact on these situations.

Q: *How does creatine help?*
A: A paper published in *Diabetes* in 2001 by Eijnde found a 40 percent increase in GLUT4 protein in the creatine group compared to the placebo group. GLUT4 is instrumental in enabling insulin to transport blood sugar into the cells.

In addition, we have already mentioned studies showing that creatine reduces triglyceride levels and total cholesterol levels. This evidence shows that creatine improves insulin sensitivity and reduces insulin resistance.

Another line of evidence is that creatine increases muscle glycogen levels, since glycogen production is dependent on insulin action. So I believe that the insulin has to be working more efficiently in order to produce a greater synthesis of glycogen. Finally, a study published in the *Journal of Applied Physiology* in 2003 found that when resistance training was combined with a creatine and protein supplement, glucose tolerance improved.

Q: *You previously mentioned the possibility that creatine has a positive impact on levels of homocysteine (a toxic amino acid linked to many age-related disorders). Could that have anti-aging properties?*

A: There is a strong possibility that creatine could provide an anti-aging effect because of its impact on homocysteine levels. Although studies are conflicting, there is one animal study showing that creatine supplementation reduced homocysteine levels. We will have to wait for more studies in order to be certain about how creatine impacts homocysteine in humans.

Q: *What about creatine and brain function? Is there any evidence that creatine helps to maintain mental faculties as we grow older?*

A: That is a very interesting area and yes, it does appear that creatine has a positive impact on brain function. There are studies showing that creatine provides protection for nerve tissue, which includes the brain. In animal studies, creatine offers protection against the equivalent of Alzheimer's disease, Parkinson's disease, Huntington's disease, amyotrophic lateral sclerosis, and others.

For example, in one animal study published in *Neurology* in 2000, it was found that creatine reduced traumatic brain damage by 36 percent in mice and 50 percent in rats. The protection appeared to be related to maintenance of mitochondrial bioenergetics and reduced free radical levels.

ATP (adenosine triphosphate) protects tissues from the damage that results when there is a reduction in oxygen, and as you will recall, creatine helps maintain ATP levels. So in essence, creatine helps to protect nerve tissue when there is a reduction in blood supply, which is what happens with stroke. Animal studies have also found creatine to protect the brain from toxins.

Creatine has also been shown to improve oxygen utilization by the brain and to reduce mental fatigue, something that could greatly benefit us as we get older. So creatine is good for the muscle in your head, as well as the muscles in the rest of your body!

Q: What are some of the things people can do to prevent signs of aging?
A: There is a wide variety of approaches to the aging process. I advocate a comprehensive scientific approach using laboratory evaluations. There are some amazing tests available now, including those that can identify your genetic makeup as related to different areas of your health.

For instance, there are cardiovascular profiles, osteoporosis profiles, and immune profiles. You can have an analysis of your DNA to see if you have any susceptibility to different metabolic abnormalities or imperfections that can be modified with proper intervention.

Q: What kinds of intervention can be of help?
A: Usually, we prescribe specific diets, nutritional supplements, and lifestyle changes, including exercise.

Q: What are some of the factors that can be modified?
A: One is oxidative stress or free radical activity, and that is associated mostly with impaired mitochondrial function. Mitochondria produce most of the free radicals in the body and if there is an excess of free radical production, it is probably related to the mitochondria not functioning properly—in other

words, not producing energy efficiently. So that is one area that can be investigated.

Other areas are carbohydrate metabolism, chronic inflammation, nutrient insufficiencies, impaired detoxification capacity, poor immune function, chronic stress response, and hormonal imbalances.

Q: And all these can be identified with lab tests?
A: There are laboratory tests that can be done to investigate all these mechanisms of unhealthy aging.

Q: What happens after lab test results are obtained?
A: Each individual can have a customized plan consisting of diet, nutritional supplementation, and other therapies, such as stress reduction, metabolic detoxification, immune stimulation, hormone replacement, or medication, in order to reduce the processes that accelerate unhealthy aging.

And of course, exercise is key. I feel weight training is even more important than aerobic training, especially for older people. That is not to say that people should not do cardiovascular exercise, but weight training is where the focus should be for people who want to remain healthy as they age. They need to work on strength and muscle, and creatine should be a part of that effort.

Q: Does this approach work for everyone?
A: Yes, to some degree. Remember that we are unique individuals and the effects of any program will be different for each person. But I think everyone will benefit in some way.

Q: How do you know when the program is working for you?
A: You can have your biomarkers tested—you can have measurements taken to which a biological age can be assigned. Some

of the biomarkers I test are muscle mass, body fat percentage, intracellular water percentage, strength, blood pressure, breathing capacity, and range of motion. All these factors can be measured against the average by age group.

Q: Can you give an example?
A: You can measure someone's intracellular water percentage and if it comes out to 65 percent, that is the average for a thirty-year-old. If the person I am testing is actually forty years old, that is a very nice result! You have a biomarker that is much younger than your chronological age. Then you can be retested every few months to see what kind of progress you are making.

Q: What is your opinion of the theory that eating very little, almost to the point of starvation, can lengthen our lives?
A: Calorie restriction has been found, at least in animal studies, to produce a dramatic increase in longevity and health. The animals are probably not too happy about going hungry, but they are healthier and live up to 50 percent longer. That is a dramatic difference.

There are no similar studies in people, but I think it is likely that calorie restriction will have a similar impact on human health. Of course, there are people who are already living this way and have been for many years.

Q: What is the evidence that calorie restriction prolongs life?
A: With aging, genes that are associated with stress and damage to the tissues are turned on and genes that repair tissues are turned off. With calorie restriction, however, you see largely the opposite: the stress genes are shut off and the repair genes are turned on.

Q: *Do you advocate this approach to anti-aging?*

A: I do advocate curtailing caloric intake, but this degree of calorie restriction is fairly extreme and would not appeal to most people. There may also be long-term unwanted side effects that we don't know about yet. I think that there might be other ways to get similar results. There may be other methods to achieve optimal energy production within the mitochondria without excessive production of free radicals, and also to normalize swings in the hormones that occur with excessive eating. So if you modify your diet, lifestyle and exercise, and take the right supplements for your individual needs, you can achieve a more optimal hormonal balance.

Hormones including insulin, respond to diet and lifestyle. So by using a natural approach, we can help optimize the biochemicals that are playing a role in the benefits of calorie restriction and perhaps get similar benefits without starving.

Points to Remember

- The signs of aging are not inevitable, and we can take steps to reverse them.
- Many signs of aging are associated with free radical damage.
- Antioxidants combat free radicals and creatine has antioxidant properties.
- Loss of muscle mass and strength are two major signs of aging, and creatine helps to reverse both.
- Creatine increases intracellular water, which helps maintain strength in the cells.
- Creatine also decreases high cholesterol and triglyceride levels, which are linked to many age-related health problems.
- Insulin resistance, linked to many age-related health conditions, appears to improve with creatine.

- Creatine protects nerve tissue, including the brain, and helps to maintain good mental function.
- Laboratory tests can provide important clues for an individualized anti-aging program.
- Calorie restriction may prolong life, but other less severe approaches may provide similar benefits.

CHAPTER TWELVE

Dr. Debé's Program for Better Sports Performance and Better Health

BY NOW, YOU have learned a great deal about creatine, your body, maximal sports performance, and enhanced health. Today, there is so much information available that it is easy to become confused and overwhelmed. How do you put it all together? And exactly what is right for you and your needs? In this chapter, you will learn how to maximize your sports performance and stay healthy.

DIET

Some of the areas that people need to consider in regard to diet and sports performance are water, carbohydrates, proteins, fats, vitamins, minerals, and phytonutrients.

Water and Liquids: It is very important to consume sufficient water on a daily basis. For an average sized person, the usual recommendation is eight 8-ounce glasses of water per day, but athletes usually need more.

If you are an athlete exercising and sweating heavily, it is important that afterward you drink two 8-ounce glasses of water for every pound of weight lost during activity. In that way, you can replace the lost water immediately after the exercise or competition. Athletes should also drink water during their workouts. And if the workout produces a lot of sweating, particularly if it's a lengthy workout that lasts longer than an hour, they can also use a good electrolyte drink that contains sodium, chloride, potassium, magnesium, and some carbohydrates.

The quality of the water is also important. I recommend drinking water that is as pure as possible as often as you can. Water should not have chlorine or other toxins in it. Most public water supplies are chlorinated in order to kill off dangerous organisms, but chlorine is not a good substance to ingest. I recommend using filtered water.

The water you bathe in is also important, so I recommend that if possible, the entire water system in your home be filtered. That will remove impurities from the water that enter your skin and that you inhale while bathing. Reverse osmosis appears to work best as a filtration system; as a second choice, carbon filtration is also effective.

Carbohydrates: There are various types of carbohydrates. Different types of carbohydrates have different effects on the body and on each individual and in each different circumstance. As a rule, it is good to eat mainly complex carbohydrates, which are long chains of sugars that require digestion for their absorption; these are usually converted to blood sugar slowly.

Simple carbohydrates are simple sugars or molecules of two sugars, which are absorbed pretty quickly and raise blood sugar very rapidly, which is usually not healthy.

Complex carbohydrates are basically whole foods that are supplied the way they are grown in nature. Brown rice is a complex carbohydrate, while white rice is refined and more of a simple carbohydrate. Vegetables and most fruits have healthy carbohydrate contents.

Fiber is another type of carbohydrate, a kind that we don't digest. Even so, the fiber in our diet has a beneficial effect in slowing absorption of blood sugar and helping the function of the gastrointestinal tract.

Lentils and legumes have a good amount of complex carbohydrates, while fruit sugars are simple. Table sugar and milk sugar are also simple carbohydrates, as are many of the sugars that are added to processed foods, such as cookies, cakes, and muffins. Another point to remember is that while fruit juice has some beneficial properties, it is also loaded with simple sugars. If you drink a lot of fruit juice quickly, you can have a fairly rapid rise in blood sugar, which for some people can negatively impact their health.

A rapid rise in blood sugar causes the release of a lot of insulin; the insulin lowers the blood sugar effectively; then other hormones are released to raise blood sugar levels. Cortisol, epinephrine, norepinephrine, glucagon, and growth hormone can all rise when people consume a lot of simple sugars, causing an unhealthy fluctuation in hormones, which can accelerate the aging process.

People respond differently to these surges. A young, lean athlete with a lot of muscle mass who has good insulin sensitivity can probably handle a surge in blood sugar much better than an elderly, sedentary individual with low muscle mass, obesity, and diabetes. The latter individual would have a lot more negative health consequences from a surge in blood sugar.

Before, during and after exercise is the most appropriate time to consume simple carbohydrates. They help to prolong aerobic exercise, replenish glycogen stores, and increase nutrient transport into cells. But no matter who you are, having too many simple sugars in your diet is definitely not good for your health.

Whole Foods: In general, the diet should consist mostly of whole foods, largely unrefined, the way nature provides them. That means vegetables, beans, nuts, seeds, fruits, animal products, meat, and grain, and all of these without excessive processing. You should try to avoid food that has its fiber, vitamins, and minerals stripped away and artificial ingredients added.

Of course, you can eat just about anything once in a while. I think people should enjoy themselves and treat themselves to whatever foods they like from time to time. But if half of your diet is made up of soda and ice cream, you are not going to be too healthy for long. So junk food can be eaten occasionally, but it should be kept to a minimum.

I don't think it's good for people to feel constantly deprived. Some athletes are prone to eating disorders, and if people restrict themselves too much, they are also more likely to wind up going on eating binges and consuming excessive quantities of the wrong things. Moderation is really the key.

Protein: In most cases, the range of protein that is appropriate for an athlete is between 1.3 and 1.8 grams of protein per kilogram of body weight (which is equivalent to about 2.2 pounds of body weight), probably toward the upper range for strength athletes. For most Americans, their regular diet usually supplies these protein levels, so there is normally no need to use supplements.

Even so, many athletes regularly use protein supplements. I am not opposed to it, but I also observe many strength athletes going overboard on protein. They think that they need much more protein than they actually do and wind up consuming it in excessive levels. They have the mindset that "more is better." What they don't realize is that too much protein can have a negative effect on the body. It can result in excessive ammonia levels, which the body has to detoxify and which can also cause headaches and other symptoms.

If you eat too much protein at one time, it can't be completely digested and absorbed. It then becomes food for unfriendly bacteria in the intestinal tract. Many people don't realize that we have 100 trillion bacteria living in our intestines. When our bodies are in balance, everything is fine. But it is very easy for the flora to become imbalanced, which can happen from poor diet, stress, or the use of antibiotics. Antibiotics can kill off friendly strains of bacteria and permit unfriendly organisms to proliferate. Eating too much protein can cause an overgrowth in certain bacteria that may have negative health consequences, including links to colon cancer.

A high-protein, low-fiber diet can also increase the number of specific bacteria in the intestinal tract that produce enzymes that are responsible for the recirculation of waste products from the intestines back into the bloodstream. Since these bacteria are stimulated by meat, a high-meat diet can accelerate the activity of these bacteria, with the end result that toxins are not eliminated, but are made into a reabsorbable form, pass back into the bloodstream and continue to damage the body.

Which kind of protein is best for athletes? For muscle building, animal protein is probably best. Not only do animal proteins contain creatine, they also result in higher levels of certain anabolic hormones, insulin-like growth factor 1 and testosterone. That is not to say that vegetarians can't build muscle, just that animal proteins are more effective.

Vegetarians: It is important for vegetarians to pay special attention to their protein consumption, because different plant proteins are lacking in specific amino acids. Because of this, vegetarians need to consume complementary proteins. For example, beans and rice together will supply all the essential amino acids, as will corn and peas. This consumption of complementary proteins needs to be done within a 24-hour period, and it does not have to be done at every single meal.

Nature's Best Protein Source: To the surprise of many, the best protein source in nature is the egg. Whey protein, which is extracted from milk, may be a little better for building muscle, but the whole food protein that is the best without any kind of processing or extraction is the whole egg. Not just the egg white.

The egg white and the yolk together give the egg the best amino acid makeup for muscle building and for human protein synthesis in general. We have been told for some time to avoid the yolk because of cholesterol, but that is a myth. As far as cholesterol goes, it is important to realize that it is a misconception that eggs raise your cholesterol level. Most people have high cholesterol levels because they eat too many carbohydrates. When you increase the amount of cholesterol in your diet, your liver produces less cholesterol. A good 70 percent of the cholesterol in your bloodstream is manufactured in your liver—it does not come from your diet. Only a small percentage comes from the diet.

You can increase your blood cholesterol levels from dietary cholesterol by only about 15 percent, but you can increase them a lot more by causing an increase in your insulin levels, which helps regulate enzymes that manufacture cholesterol.

So it is not necessary to avoid eggs because you fear high blood cholesterol. Studies have found that eating eggs produces very little change in blood cholesterol levels. Not only are eggs the best protein source in nature, they also have other valuable nutrients, like high levels of choline, B vitamins and selenium. There are also several brands of eggs that are high in a beneficial omega-3 fatty acid called DHA. The eggs have DHA because the hens are fed dried algae, which has DHA that is incorporated into the eggs.

As a rule, I recommend eating a few eggs at one meal. For a large athlete, one or two may not be enough. But I believe that a few eggs a few times a week is generally a good idea. Cooking methods are important. Boiling eggs is best, while frying eggs may oxidize the cholesterol and make it toxic.

Variety: I think that variety is very important in one's diet. You can have a very healthy breakfast, a very healthy lunch, and a very healthy dinner, but if you are eating the same food in your meals day after day, you can still have problems.

You need variety for a number of reasons. First, because each food has its own strengths and weaknesses, each food has certain nutrients and is lacking in others. So if you don't have enough variety, you are more likely to be deficient in various nutrients.

The second reason is that if you are eating the same foods all the time, you are likely to develop an intolerance to these foods. One of the things that contributes to food intolerance, sensitivities or reactions is the frequency with which the food is consumed. If your immune system is exposed to the same foods day after day and in some cases, meal after meal, it is more likely to become sensitized to the food, begin to recognize the food as a foreign invader and mount an attack against it. That will produce adverse health effects. So always try to vary your foods and avoid eating the same items too often.

Fats: Fats contain compounds called fatty acids. There are two fatty acids—linoleic acid and alpha linolenic acid—that are essential, which means they cannot be manufactured in the body and must be obtained from the diet. If they are not obtained from the diet, the body's physiology is compromised and we develop symptoms of deficiency.

Linoleic acid is classified as an omega-6 fatty acid and is found in nuts, seeds, vegetables, and oils derived from these foods. Most Americans get enough linoleic acid in their diets.

Arachidonic acid, another omega-6 fatty acid, is derived from beef, lamb, pork, dairy products, eggs, shellfish, and peanuts.

Arachidonic acid is converted into inflammatory chemicals in the body, so if there is any inflammation in the body, consuming these foods is like pouring gasoline on a fire—it makes the inflammation worse. So if athletes are injured and aren't healing as rapidly as they should, or if they suffer frequent injuries, they should investigate whether they may be consuming too much arachidonic-acid rich foods.

The fatty acids that most Americans lack in their diets are omega-3 fatty acids, which are largely anti-inflammatory. They are found in soybean oil, walnut oil, canola oil, perilla seed oil, hemp seed oil, and flaxseed oil. Flaxseed oil gives us the most concentrated form of plant-derived omega-3 oils. Other omega-3 oils are found in algae and coldwater fish like ocean salmon, sardines, and mackerel. Two specific types of omega-3 fatty acids found in these fish are EPA and DHA, both of which are very important.

Many people are lacking in sufficient levels of EPA and DHA. EPA is anti-inflammatory and reduces platelet clotting, making it a kind of blood thinner. DHA is found in high concentrations in the brain and retina and is essential for nerve function. So it is important for people to examine their diets to be certain they are getting enough of these important nutrients from their food.

Saturated Fats: We also have to realize that not all fats are beneficial, and Americans are getting too much of saturated fats in their diet. They are found in such foods as butter, mayonnaise, whole fat dairy products, beef, and cheese. When it comes to beef, you are better off choosing the lowest fat cuts, like sirloin and filet mignon. You can also try other types of meat that have healthier fatty acid profiles, such as buffalo and ostrich, which can be found in many health food stores.

Your body can do without saturated fats. The body actually can manufacture saturated fats and does not need them from the diet in any major amount. But if you are eating animal products, you are definitely going to get some. That's why you need to examine your diet to be sure you are not getting an excessive amount. Saturated fats are more solid at room temperature and they are more solid in your body, as well. They can cause rigidity in cell membranes and can impair the function of cell membranes, where the transfer of nutrients and waste products occurs.

The saturated fat content of many of the foods we buy is now listed on the label. A general guideline is no more than 25 percent of your total dietary fat consumption should be saturated fat, preferably less.

Monounsaturated Fat: The body can manufacture monounsaturated fat, but it is a type of fat that people should make an effort to consume because it has some beneficial health effects. Monounsaturated fat is found in olives, olive oil, avocados, and many nuts. It has a beneficial effect on reducing inflammation and on cholesterol levels, apparently increasing beneficial HDL cholesterol.

Trans-fats: You should make an effort to reduce or preferably eliminate trans-fats from your diet. Trans-fats are even worse than saturated fats, although they are similar in structure and function. Today, the average person consumes 2,000 times more trans-fats than was consumed in 1850. Trans-fats result from heavy food processing and have many negative health effects.

They were developed years ago, when the unhealthy effects of saturated fats were discovered. Food manufacturers came up with an alternative that they thought would be better: hydrogenated vegetable oils. You can find them in all kinds of convenience foods, including chips, cake, cookies, bread, and other baked goods. Once again, you should read the labels.

The manufacturing procedure involves vegetable oils, which are polyunsaturated (and more liquid at room temperature). These vegetable oils are infused with hydrogen and become more saturated, more solid at room temperature. In the food industry, that is a benefit because the hydrogenated vegetable oils can substitute for animal-source saturated fats and also increase shelf life.

However, it has been known for several years that trans-fats are even more harmful to the body than saturated fats. They have a negative effect on blood lipids and insulin sensitivity and have been linked to other ill effects on body chemistry.

For these reasons, I recommend that people choose saturated fats over hydrogenated vegetable oils, if those are the only choices available.

Fried Foods and Oils: Try not to consume too many fried foods. When oil is heated to high temperatures, as it is during frying, the oil is damaged and becomes toxic. You also have to consider the source of the oil that is being used in cooking. Is it from a plant or an animal? What kind of fatty acids does it contain—omega-6, omega-3, saturated, or trans-fats?

When you're looking for healthy oils, you also have to know how the oil has been extracted, processed, stored and used in cooking, because the wrong treatment of oil at any one of those steps can turn a healthy oil into an unhealthy oil. For example, flaxseed oil should never be used for cooking. The oil has to be extracted in the absence of heat, light, and oxygen; it has to be stored in an opaque container without oxygen; it should not be exposed to light; and once it's open, it should be refrigerated and never heated to excessive levels. For maximum benefit, flaxseed oil should be consumed raw.

In most supermarkets, the only healthy oil you can find is olive oil. Most of the other oils on the shelf are not good for you: they are in clear bottles, they have been excessively processed, and their vitamins, minerals and phytonutrients have been removed. That may improve their shelf life, but it also produces an oil that is not good for your health.

So a supermarket is not the best place to purchase cooking oil. I do not recommend cooking with safflower oil, sunflower oil, or corn oil. But I do recommend cooking with olive oil or even butter as a second choice. And I recommend flaxseed oil and olive oil to put on salads and vegetables.

Phytonutrients, Vitamins and Minerals: Phytonutrients are plant-derived non-essential compounds that are not vitamins or minerals. There are thousands of phytonutrients and they have many beneficial effects on the human body, including protection against cancer. If you eat a whole food diet rich in plant foods that have not been processed or refined, then you will get a lot of vitamins, minerals, fiber, and other phytonutrients. But if you eat a diet that is composed of very refined foods, like white bread, bagels, pasta, and white rice, then you will miss out on a lot of these phytonutrients.

Phytonutrients include flavonoids, found in citrus fruits; indoles found in Brussels sprouts and cabbage; genistein, found in soybeans; and saponins, found in soybeans, lentils, and kidney beans. There are many others that can be found in the vegetables, fruit and grains we eat, especially if these foods are eaten raw or only minimally cooked.

Whole foods also contain a lot of beneficial vitamins and minerals. One of their important jobs is to act as coenzymes. Most of the chemical reactions that occur in the body are facilitated by special proteins called enzymes. For enzymes to function, they require coenzymes, which are usually vitamins or minerals. So if you're lacking the coenzyme necessary for a particular enzymatic reaction, then that aspect of your physiology is going to suffer.

For example, the enzyme that converts the thyroid hormone T-4 into the more active T-3 has selenium as a coenzyme. So if your diet is lacking in the mineral selenium, as many American diets are, you will not have optimal levels of the active thyroid hormone in your body.

Vitamins, which can be water-soluble or oil-soluble, are essential to life, although as micronutrients they are needed only in small amounts. Vitamins regulate metabolism and are an important component to creating energy in the body.

Like vitamins, minerals are also essential to good health and are essential to energy production, growth, healing and many other body functions. Stored in bone and muscle tissue, they are also needed only in small amounts. But a lack of needed levels of any of the essential vitamins or minerals can have serious health consequences.

Biochemical Individuality: Something else that is important is biochemical individuality. The human genome project identified over 1.4 million variations in genetic structure among individuals. So if we just focus on the enzymes, each person can have a different enzyme structure. That means that one person may have a less efficient form of an enzyme than another and in order to get a less efficient form of an enzyme to be optimally active, you need more of the coenzyme, and therefore more vitamins and minerals.

In other words, nutrient needs vary from person to person by as much as five hundred-fold or more, so we can't just go by the government's recommended dietary intakes to decide how much of each nutrient we should consume. We have to find out what each of us as individuals actually needs.

I recommend that people have a comprehensive evaluation of their nutritional status. The test I like to perform on my patients evaluates amino acids, fatty acids, vitamins, minerals, and other compounds called organic acids, which give us insights into various metabolic functions. I also evaluate free radicals and antioxidant balance. Based on this type of evaluation, each individual's nutritional needs can be better met.

So instead of guessing or treating everyone as an "average" individual, we can be scientific and determine what each individual needs for his or her body to function optimally. And I tell my patients that when we run the test, if we don't come up with some deficiency, I will pay for it myself because it is guaranteed that everyone has something that is lacking, even people who take a lot of supplements.

Eating Frequency and Caloric Requirements: I recommend that people eat their meals more frequently during the day. Ideally, you should have five meals a day, although you can eat as many meals as you like, so long as you are not eating excessively. In addition to what you eat and how often you eat, it is also important to be sure you meet your caloric requirements every day. Especially if you are an athlete and are trying to build muscle and perform at your best in your sport, you must consume adequate calories. But you also have to be certain not to overeat, since you don't want to put on excess body fat.

For building muscle, burning body fat, and lowering cholesterol levels, it is best to eat small, frequent meals. If you take the same diet you are eating and consume it in small meals spaced throughout the day, you will have a better effect on your sports performance and muscle building. It is not good to go too long without eating. So I recommend that people try to eat something about every three hours.

Caffeine: Caffeine has not been shown to directly increase strength or muscle building, and in excess, caffeine is not beneficial for health. Caffeine can increase speed and power output in activities lasting between 60 seconds and two hours, and it may be of some benefit for endurance sports. If people enjoy drinking caffeinated beverages in moderation, I don't think that is harmful for most. And moderate caffeine consumption may help protect against Parkinson's disease and colorectal cancer because it speeds up the activity of certain detoxification enzymes. That helps the body rid itself of toxins more efficiently. And as with anything else, the negative effects of caffeine will vary from person to person, depending on biochemical individuality.

Alcohol: I think that alcohol in moderation—one or two small drinks a day—is all right, but I do not recommend it for trying to improve sports performance. Alcohol does have some negative health effects, so strictly from a health point of view, it is important to evaluate each individual's needs. How you respond to alcohol can determine how beneficial or dangerous it is for you. Some people are prone to alcohol abuse and are unable to drink without drinking to excess. And in excess, alcohol is very detrimental to athletic performance, since it is toxic to striated muscle.

Tobacco: Smoking has no benefits at all when it comes to the athletic performance and health of the average person. However, it may surprise you to learn that smoking can actually have some benefits. Research shows that tobacco alters detoxification enzymes in the body and that in certain individuals, it can help people metabolize hormones in a more healthy way. There is also some evidence of a small benefit in certain autoimmune conditions.

But there are really no reasons to smoke, especially if you are interested in maximal sports performance. One study, which appeared in a 1998 issue of the *Indian Journal of Experimental Biology*, entitled "Effect of cigarette smoking on muscle strength and flexibility in athletes," examined smoking and nonsmoking athletes. The researchers found that tobacco smoke had a negative effect on both flexibility and strength.

This finding is not surprising because tobacco smoke, among other things, contains huge quantities of free radicals, which damage tissues throughout the body. So for any athlete seeking optimal performance and effective muscle building, smoking is something to avoid at all costs.

Supplements

Creatine: For strength athletes and people looking to build muscle, I recommend creatine first and foremost. Begin with a loading phase, 5 grams four times a day for five days, and then go into a maintenance phase, taking 3 to 5 grams a day. Larger, very active athletes may need a little bit more, up to 10 grams a day, but the average person should take 5 grams a day.

I also recommend that athletes consider cycling the creatine, possibly taking it for eight weeks, then having a break for two to four weeks and then going through a loading phase again. It is also a good idea to go through a loading phase just before a competition.

Whey Protein and Carbohydrate: I recommend a combination of protein and carbohydrate before and after workouts. One of the best protein sources is whey; others to consider are egg and casein. Vegetarians can use soy, and there are some soy proteins that are fortified with methionine to complete the amino acid profile. There are also other vegetable proteins that can be used.

Before a workout, I recommend 10 to 20 grams of protein with 50 to 60 grams of carbohydrate. After a workout, I recom-

John: Building Muscle at Last

John, a 45-year-old real estate salesman, consulted me because he was interested in gaining weight, improving his energy and mood and lowering his cholesterol levels. Although John appeared to be healthy and fit, he was definitely too thin. In fact, he told me he had always been underweight, and it had always been a problem for him.

John was on a good weight training exercise program, but his diet was poor. After doing a workup, I encouraged John to eat more frequently and also educated him regarding the truth about eating eggs. John, like most people, thought that eating eggs would raise his bad cholesterol levels, so he avoided them. I explained that for most people, eggs do not have an adverse effect on blood cholesterol levels or heart disease, and that eggs are the best complete protein found in nature. Since John was not eating enough and needed more protein to build muscle, I recommended that he begin eating some eggs.

Laboratory tests revealed that John had elevated cortisol and abnormally low levels of DHEA, two important hormones. Since high levels of cortisol result in reduced protein synthesis and accelerated protein breakdown and low DHEA levels result in an inability to combat the negative effects of high cortisol, John's body was working against his desire to gain muscle, strength, and body weight.

I felt that John's poor diet, especially the low protein content, was one of the major reasons for his imbalanced levels of cortisol and DHEA. The elevated cortisol to DHEA ratio could also be the cause of John's fatigue, depression and elevated blood cholesterol levels.

I prescribed DHEA supplements, as well as phosphorylated serine to help John lower his cortisol levels. He also began taking a stress adaptogenic formula containing Korean ginseng, cordyceps, and rhodiola; and whey protein mixed with water, frozen berries and a formula containing creatine monohydrate, glutamine, taurine and HMB. The whey protein mixture was consumed as a snack between meals, twice a day.

Other changes to John's diet included increasing his intake of vegetables and the addition of sardines and salmon.

John had great results on this program, gaining 5 pounds in just one month. He also saw improvements in energy, mood, sleep patterns, and an overall sense of well-being. John told me that he felt stronger and his friends and family were telling him that he looked much younger.

A follow-up stress hormone test two months later found that John's cortisol and DHEA levels were now in the normal range. We gradually tapered off on the DHEA and phosphorylated serine supplements, but John continues using the other supplements and sticking to his diet plan. In a short time, we will check his cholesterol levels, and I feel certain that he will show progress in this area as well.

mend 15 to 50 grams of protein and 50 to 120 grams of carbohydrate. But these recommendations are not going to apply to everyone, especially when it comes to the carbohydrates.

People who have carbohydrate metabolism problems, whether they know it or not, must be very cautious about using that amount of carbohydrate. And diabetics already know they will have problems with those levels of carbohydrate, so they can't take that much. Other people who have carbohydrate metabolism problems and may not know it are those with insulin resistance that results in obesity, hypertension, high cholesterol levels, and high triglyceride levels.

Others who have to watch their carbohydrate intake are those with increased waist measurements of over 40 inches in men and 34 inches in women, as well as an elevated waist-hip ratio. If you measure your waist around the belly button and then your hips at their widest point around the buttocks, then divide the waist measurement by the hip measurement and the number is over .95 in men and .80 in women, that is consistent with insulin metabolism problems.

Of course, if you have elevated insulin or glucose levels on blood testing, that is also a sign of these problems. In general, the elderly are more prone to these problems. All the people who fall into this category need to be more cautious about using carbohydrates and should discuss this with a qualified health care professional.

HMB: For strength and increasing fat free mass, HMB is a good supplement to consider. The research so far does not show that it is as effective as creatine, but there is some evidence that it can be helpful to certain individuals. One drawback is the price and another is taking 12 capsules a day. However, HMB is also available in powder form, combined with creatine. If you want to get an additional edge, HMB is worth a try. The dosage used in studies is 3 grams a day, which is 4 capsules three times a day.

Adaptogens: I also recommend that athletes in heavy training consider using adaptogens, which are compounds that help the body to adapt to stress and withstand it more effectively. That includes the physical stress of heavy exercise training. Three of the best adaptogens are the herbs Korean ginseng, cordyceps, and rhodiola. It is very important that these herbs be of the highest quality, so those who want to try them should consult a knowledgeable health care professional or herbalist before buying.

Most people are familiar with ginseng, which has been used in Asia for centuries as a stimulant for both mental and physical activities. It enhances athletic performance by sparing glycogen and stimulating the use of fatty acids for energy. Ginseng is available in many forms, including whole root, root pieces, powder, capsules, tablets, and tea.

Cordyceps is derived from a type of mushroom and has been shown to improve aerobic capacity in athletes. There is also research showing benefits on different organ systems and metabolic functions, including glucose and lipid metabolism. Cordyceps has traditionally been used to help support the body after exhaustion.

Rhodiola comes from Eastern Europe and Asia and is also known as "Arctic root." It has traditionally been used to promote stamina and energy and enhance physical and mental performance. Rhodiola has been used widely by Russian athletes.

Supplement Use: In general, I recommend taking vitamin and mineral supplements and other nutrients that are found to be lacking with a scientific assessment of each individual. Most people will derive health benefits from supplements of vitamin C and vitamin E, although it is not likely that these supplements will increase strength or muscle mass directly. But they may benefit indirectly, as may other supplements, because they can help keep an athlete healthy and in regular training. If you are ill and miss regular training, you will have a hard time reaching the ultimate performance that you could have reached if you had remained healthy.

Exercise

Athletes need to do sport-specific exercise, and people who use creatine range from non-athletes all the way to world-champion athletes. These people have different degrees of familiarity with exercise, but seasoned athletes should be working with a strength and conditioning coach who can help them achieve peak physical condition.

To start off, we can give some general recommendations. For people over forty and for anyone with less than perfect health, it is a good idea to consult a doctor and have a thorough physical examination before beginning an exercise program.

Weight training is the most effective way to strengthen and build muscle. It is done with weight machines and free weights. For the beginner, weight machines are usually an easier way to become accustomed to the exercise. There is less of a chance of injury and it is easier to master the movements than with free barbells or dumbbells.

For beginners, I recommend starting off with training three times a week. Initially, it is probably a good idea to work with someone who is knowledgeable—a personal trainer or other professional. In the beginning, your efforts should be slight, since you need time to become familiar with the exercise. But after only a few weeks of training, you should be pushing yourself hard, although you should never sacrifice form at the expense of completing a repetition.

When we talk about weight training, there are many different exercises that can be done. For most individuals, the exercises that produce the greatest payoff are exercises that work large muscle groups and multiple joints at the same time. These exercises include the leg press or barbell squat, for the lower extremities—legs and hips; the bench press or chest fly for the pectoralis or chest muscles; and what we call the "lat pull down" for muscles in the upper back.

Those are three of the more important exercises because they work the largest muscle groups in the body at one time. In addition to whatever else you do, it is always a good idea to be certain you are doing exercises that work multiple joints at once and that do not overly isolate muscle groups. Muscle isolation is not as effective as more whole body exercises.

After training with weights for a period of time, your goal should be to work to failure on each set of repetitions. A set refers to the time frame in which you engage in a series of lifts. For weight training and for strengthening muscle, the number of repetitions or lifts should be about eight to twelve. Of course, if you are a power lifter or weight lifter, you will have your own routines to follow and will typically use lower repetitions. But for most strength athletes, eight to twelve reps is usually a good range.

As to the number of sets, there is some debate on how many sets are optimal. Three sets is often recommended as a good number per exercise. A recent study found that doing one set of an exercise gave about 98 percent of the benefits of three sets. So there is really no excuse for people not to do some weight training because of time constraints. I have had very good workouts in under fifteen minutes. I just target a few of the large muscle group exercises and do one set each. In that way, I can accomplish a lot in just a few minutes. So if you don't have a lot of time to devote to exercise, working hard with just one set on each exercise can still produce good results.

Another consideration in weight training is how long to rest between sets or between exercises (see below). You don't want to push yourself to exhaustion initially, but after you've been working for a few weeks, you should be striving to have a very short rest period between exercises, probably about a minute or less.

Another important consideration is to vary your exercises over time. You don't want to do the same exercises indefinitely; you want to add some variety to the routine to keep it interesting and also to challenge your muscles more effectively. If you do the same exercises over and over again, your muscles will adapt to them to the extent that they may not give you the results you want. Remember that your muscles grow by stressing them, actually causing micro-injuries with the exercise, and then allowing them to rest, recover and grow bigger and stronger in response to the stress.

If bigger and stronger muscles were produced simply by a lot of activity, then mailmen would be the strongest people in the world because of the amount of exercise they get. But the amount is not the only factor. It's important that the exercise be maximal and progressive. So when you lift a weight today and go all out and do as much as you can, if you only do that over and over and nothing more, your body will adapt to it and will not grow and become stronger.

Therefore, you need to regularly strive to increase the weight, the repetitions and/or the number of sets and reduce the rest time between exercises or sets in order to make it more challenging for your body and cause the proper response to achieve the results you want.

Even people who can't use weights can benefit from strength training by other methods. I think weights are ideal, but people who don't have access to weights can strengthen their bodies with calisthenics, for example, using their body weight for resistance. They can do exercises like chin-ups or push-ups.

There are also devices that may be more accessible and portable than weights, like resistance bands, which are elastic tubes that can be secured on one end and then pulled with an arm or leg to strengthen the body.

People who are in poor physical condition, like many of the institutionalized elderly, can begin with just manual resistance. You have another individual push against the body part as the person doing the exercise exerts force and tries to push or pull a limb. Of course, you should only do exercises like that with someone who is trained and knows precisely how to do these exercises safely, to avoid any possibility of injury.

For someone who doesn't have access to anything else, the light resistance of holding a can of food or a light, hand-held dumbbell weighing one or two pounds, is better than nothing. That is fine for a beginning. But once that is accomplished with ease, you need to increase the resistance in order to get results.

Rest

In order for muscles to grow bigger and stronger, they need a rest period after strenuous workouts. Initially, people should probably start out with only three weight training sessions per week. In addition to resting between workouts, nighttime sleep needs to be adequate. Everyone varies in the amount of sleep that they need, but eight hours is a number that is a good goal for most people. And it is not only the number of hours that you spend in bed. The sleep must be deep, restful, and restorative and if it is not, that should be evaluated by a health care professional to determine the reason.

Sometimes poor quality sleep is a result of stress or excessive use of caffeine. It can also be a sign of over-training.

Many people benefit from taking a short nap in the afternoon if it's possible to fit that into your lifestyle. Twenty minutes or more of sleep in mid-afternoon helps to rejuvenate energy, including mental capacity. And it also relieves the effects of gravity on the body for a period of time, which helps to repair the joints.

I recommend taking off at least one day a week from exercise training. This is important for everyone, but especially for the many athletes who have a tendency toward over-training. It's very easy to get overzealous about an exercise and sports program and work too hard at it. Believe it or not, that can actually give you worse results.

If you don't give your body enough time to rest and heal, you are not going to have the increases in strength and muscle mass that you want. Some of the signs of over-training are the following: poor quality sleep, fatigue, changes in mood, increased susceptibility to infections, and an increase in the heart rate, especially upon waking in the morning. There are also some laboratory tests that can be done to look for biochemical signs that an athlete might be over-training.

In addition to adequate, quality rest, stress-reduction is something that is important for many people. It can actually be very helpful with training. There are many different approaches to stress-reduction and each person needs to find the one that works for her or him. They include massage, yoga, meditation, guided imagery, deep breathing exercises, and relaxing herbs such as valerian root, passion flower, and skullcap.

Injury Prevention

Any athlete or anyone looking to excel in sports or improve body composition needs regular training, that is, consistent exercise. Obviously, if you are troubled by severe or repetitive injuries, you are not going to do as well as you could if you remained healthy and injury-free. There are some steps people can take to be pro-active and avoid injuries in the first place, or at least reduce the severity of injuries when they do occur and help them heal more quickly.

First, there are a few nutritional supplements that can help. Athletes often use non-steroidal anti-inflammatory drugs prior to workouts and competitions. Not only do these drugs carry a risk of causing damage and ulceration in the gastrointestinal tract among other systemic effects, a recent study also found that these types of medications reduce protein synthesis, which is not good for anyone seeking to build muscle. And there is also evidence that these medications reduce the strength of healing tissues after injuries.

But there are alternatives that can be used to prevent injuries or to help them heal more quickly when they occur. The supplements with the most research in this regard are proteolytic enzymes.

"Proteolytic" refers to protein-splitting. These are enzymes derived from plant and animal sources that are available in supplemental capsules or tablets. When they are taken with meals, they help digest food. But to get the effect of preventing or helping heal injuries, they need to be taken between meals on an empty stomach. Then they have the effect of breaking down proteins systemically and the proteins they work on are basically tissue debris.

When there is an injury, there is a breakdown of tissue with damaged cells that rupture. The quicker that damage can be cleaned up, the quicker the healing process gets under way, and the healthier the injured tissue will eventually become.

There have been quite a few studies on the use of proteolytic enzymes prior to athletic activity, including competition in various sports such as football and boxing. These studies found that there is a significant reduction in the incidence of injury when proteolytic enzymes are used. And the injuries that are sustained are less severe and heal more rapidly. So these compounds can be used prophylactically to prevent injury and also to help injuries heal more quickly and effectively.

There have also been studies on bioflavonoids that have shown similar results. You can find supplements that combine proteolytic enzymes with bioflavonoids. Another beneficial supplement is glucosamine and chondroitin sulfate, especially for athletes who have joint injuries affecting the cartilage, tendons, and ligaments. Of course, you have to be evaluated first by a health care professional to find out exactly what your injury is and what supplements will be helpful.

When it comes to avoiding injury, one of the important things to do is to stretch before and after exercise. I recommend starting off with a six-minute aerobic exercise warmup, such as walking, cycling, or jumping rope. Then do your stretching. Additional therapies can also be helpful in injury prevention, including massage and chiropractic. Massage keeps muscles loose and flexible. Chiropractic keeps joints moving freely and studies have shown that it also improves joint range of motion, immune function and cortisol levels. And finally, getting customized foot orthotics for athletic shoes can also help to prevent injuries.

Laboratory Tests

In order to build muscle, you need not only creatine and protein and other vital nutrients, you also need to have optimal physiology. One factor that is particularly important is good insulin sensitivity. The cells need to respond to insulin's signals efficiently because insulin is an anabolic muscle-building hormone and when insulin isn't working properly, the body can't build muscle well.

For example, I recently worked with a former world-class athlete who discovered he had lost 30 pounds in a month. Tests found that he was diabetic, which is on the worst end of the continuum of insulin sensitivity. Without his body's insulin working effectively, his body was not in an anabolic state and he was not able to rebuild muscle after the muscle breakdown that occurs with training and with life in general.

So insulin sensitivity is critical for building muscle and we can best measure an individual's degree of insulin sensitivity with a carbohydrate challenge test. This test, which assesses glucose and insulin levels, requires a blood sample drawn in the morning while fasting. Then the person being tested gets a high carbohydrate meal, and during the following three hours, four more blood samples are taken and tested for glucose and insulin. The fluctuations in blood sugar and insulin are analyzed, and the results can indicate how well insulin is working in the body. The results can be used to design a healthy dietary, nutritional supplement, and lifestyle program to improve the way insulin works in the body and to lead to a more anabolic physiology.

Something else that is important for muscle building is good mitochondrial ATP production. Protein synthesis requires a lot of energy and most of that energy comes from food being burned with oxygen in the mitochondria of the cells. If these mitochondria aren't working up to par, then protein synthesis and muscle building is impaired.

There is a laboratory test called a urine organic acid analysis that gives us insight into how well the mitochondria are functioning. This test measures biochemicals which are created in the Krebs cycle or the citric acid cycle, which is the process of food being broken down in the mitochondria on its way to producing ATP. Any abnormalities in these different organic acids, such as high or low levels, can point to blocks in cellular energy production. When that is found, we can intervene with specific nutrients to help optimize energy production.

Another important factor for muscle building is to have enough of the anabolic hormones, including DHEA and testosterone. These hormones can be assessed with an analysis of a saliva specimen. Biologically active hormones are assessed best from saliva because in the blood, most of the hormone is bound to proteins and is inactive. But the hormones that pass from the blood through the salivary glands and into saliva are mostly free, unbound hormones. These hormones escape the bloodstream and make their way into the tissues to produce the effect that the hormone has on the body.

When these hormone levels are measured and you find low levels of anabolic hormones, you might use a natural, holistic approach to try to get the body to produce more of the hormones on its own. Or you may have to use a medical therapy, either by using hormone replacement or a medication that will cause increased production of the hormone in the body. Medical interventions like these are more common in older people.

Another consideration for building muscle is the balance of

catabolic hormones, the hormones that cause muscle protein breakdown. We need to have some of these hormones in our bodies, since they have beneficial effects, including helping us respond successfully to stress. It can be detrimental if we do not have sufficient levels of catabolic hormones. But when catabolic hormones are overproduced, there are many negative consequences for our health. The entire body becomes catabolic, in a state of breaking down. Muscle tissue breaks down, and protein synthesis and muscle building do not proceed normally.

One of the most important hormones in this regard is the stress hormone cortisol, which is produced by the adrenal glands. The best way to measure cortisol levels is with a saliva test. There is a test that uses four saliva specimens collected over the course of a day, because cortisol has a normal diurnal rhythm, whereby normally, levels are highest in the morning and lowest at midnight.

But with chronic stress of any type, cortisol levels can become elevated. It is particularly troubling when cortisol levels are elevated at midnight because the body does most of its repair and growth at night when we are sleeping. So if your cortisol levels are elevated then, it can interfere with growth hormone release and REM sleep, and your body can't regenerate physically or mentally.

Cortisol becomes elevated in response to stress. When most people think of stress, they think of mental or emotional stress. But anything that moves the body from equilibrium is a stress. The body responds to all stresses in the same way, with an increase in cortisol. Some types of stress that often affect athletes include over-training, heavy exercise training, swings in blood sugar, and inflammation or damage to tissues.

If a test is run and cortisol is found to be high, steps can be taken to bring it back to a more normal level. Then you will have a better chance of building muscle and strength more efficiently.

The adrenal stress index is a test that examines saliva specimens for levels of the two long-acting stress hormones, cortisol and DHEA. When people are under prolonged stress, these two hormones can be imbalanced. When you have a high cortisol-DHEA ratio, that can result in catabolic physiology, where the body's tissues are breaking down. Naturally, that is not good for anyone, especially athletes. With the adrenal stress index, we can see if that is occurring and if so, steps can be taken to balance these hormones and make the physiology more anabolic and conducive to muscle building and strengthening. That usually involves a combination of dietary changes, lifestyle changes (including increased rest and stress reduction), nutritional supplements, and sometimes exercise, as well.

Another useful test is an ION profile, which stands for "individualized optimal nutrition" profile. It is done from a combination of blood and urine specimens and measures levels of vitamins, minerals, amino acids, fatty acids, and organic acids, which are compounds produced in the course of metabolism. Based on this assessment, an athlete's nutritional needs can be identified and met.

People are often referred to recommended dietary intake (RDI) levels, but those are just the best-guess levels that are good for a number of people. There really is no average person. Everyone has different needs for given nutrients and the only way to determine what your needs are is with this type of scientific evaluation.

Testing for food sensitivities is also extremely important, and here the ALCAT test can be very helpful. This is just one type of test for food sensitivities, and there are others as well. Food sensitivity tests, using blood specimens, identify intolerances to specific foods, which are often hidden and unknown. For example, you can eat a food on Monday and not have an adverse reaction to it until Thursday. And that adverse reaction can take the form of almost any symptom you can imagine. Fatigue is one of the most common.

When you have delayed reactions like this, it is almost impossible to make an association between the offending food and the symptoms. There have been reports of world-class athletes improving their performances when hidden food sensitivities were discovered and these foods eliminated from their diets.

Another consideration with regard to muscle building is the level of catabolic inflammatory cytokines. Cytokines are immune system proteins and if your body is producing too much of certain of these inflammatory proteins, it can interfere with muscle building and cause muscle breakdown.

These inflammatory proteins can be measured from blood specimens. If they are elevated, the reason should be sought out. Some common causes include infections with different organisms and impaired function of various metabolic processes including insulin sensitivity. Once the cause is identified, there are nutritional approaches that can help to lower these compounds.

Another useful test is a comprehensive digestive analysis. If people are not digesting and absorbing nutrients properly, they are not going to be as healthy as they could be, even if they are eating a good diet. Absorption and digestion of food determine how well nutrients are actually used, and this test can provide important information in that regard.

Overall, when we look at some of the causative factors that disturb the body's physiology and interfere with muscle building, we see the following:

- nutrient deficiencies
- inadequate meal frequency
- not eating enough
- numerous varieties of stress, including mental, physical and

emotional
- inadequate or excessive exercise
- toxicity
- infections
- swings in blood sugar
- insufficient rest

Each person is a unique individual with a unique genetic makeup and biochemistry. At different points in time, people have different aberrations in their metabolic functions. So by having an individualized workup using various laboratory tests, different aspects of your physiology can be evaluated to see how well your body is working and how its functions can be optimized.

This type of evaluation is not routinely done with conventional medicine. What we are talking about here is a different approach called "functional medicine." Functional medicine strives to improve the way physiology works and prevent illness from happening in the first place, rather than being merely reactive and dealing with illness or disease after it has developed.

So I believe that everyone can benefit from these individualized types of assessments and therefore recommend that everyone who is looking for optimal health and maximal athletic performance consider having this type of individualized analysis and customized health and exercise program.

CHAPTER THIRTEEN

Conclusion

BY NOW, YOU have learned a great deal about how your body works, how energy is generated, how strength and muscle can increase, how creatine can help build muscle and strength, how other supplements may or may not be appropriate for athletes, and how you can develop a total program to maximize your athletic performance and build good health for now and the future. In this chapter, we will summarize some of the most significant things we have covered in this book.

Q: What are some of the most important points that people need to know about supplemental creatine?
A: Number one, that it works. Unlike a lot of supplements that are purported to improve sports performance, increase strength or build muscle, creatine actually does these things. There is a tremendous amount of scientific research backing this conclusion. The vast number of studies have found creatine to be effective in increasing strength and building muscle.

Number two, people need to know what types of activities and sports are best helped by creatine supplements, and those activities are the ones of short duration and high intensity.

Number three, people should know that creatine is safe. Studies evaluating the safety of creatine have consistently found that it is free of adverse side effects.

Q: Can you summarize the role of health care professionals for people who want to use creatine?
A: There is a very small possibility that an individual should not take creatine, so it is important to find out if it is safe for you. To determine that, it is best to consult a qualified, knowledgeable health care professional. A medical history, thorough examination and any necessary tests can help to find out if creatine would be a safe supplement to use, whether it should be monitored, or whether a given individual should not use it.

Health care professionals can also help by guiding the use of creatine in order to maximize its effectiveness. In that way, each person can discover how to use creatine supplements to help his or her own individual needs.

Q: How can people stay informed about the latest findings on creatine and other sports supplements and is that important?
A: If you have a bit of a scientific background and know how to read medical studies, MedLine (on the internet) is a good way to keep up-to-date on scientific findings related to sports supplements. MedLine is a service of the National Library of Medicine and has abstracts of studies from refereed peer-reviewed medical and scientific journals.

It's important to know you can be confident that the information you get from MedLine is reliable, as opposed to some of the information you may get from popular magazines or other sources, where there may be a commercial motivation to promote products.

When it comes to sports supplements, consumers have to be careful. There is a lot of hype in advertisements and articles. If you want to follow up on some of the ads, you can request published studies from the manufacturers, but they don't always respond.

It is important to stay informed about supplements because there is always the possibility that longer-term studies will discover adverse effects that were not previously known. Continued research can also come up with new ways to use supplements or reveal additional benefits that were not known before. So keeping up with research can bring you both positive and negative information that can have a significant effect on your personal supplement use.

Q: What is the best way to use supplements?
A: The best approach to supplements is to be as scientific as possible about them. When it comes to creatine, there aren't any easily accessible tests to determine whether you need supplements or how likely it is that you will respond to them. But with creatine, most people seem to have beneficial results.

With other supplements, evaluation with laboratory tests can often help to tailor an individual regimen suited to your needs. So the best way to use supplements is to find out exactly what you need, what will benefit you and what is safe for you to use. When it comes to strength building supplements, nothing works better than creatine.

Q: What should people do if the supplements they are using don't seem to work or appear to be causing health problems?
A: If your supplements do not seem to be effective or if you are experiencing side effects that you think are connected to their use, you should immediately consult a doctor or other health care professional. If you are experiencing side effects, you need to find out if they are connected to the supplement. If the sup-

plement doesn't seem to be working, there could be something wrong with the specific product you have chosen or how you are using it. For example, it could be of low quality or perhaps you are not taking the right amount or using it frequently enough. Or there could be something wrong with your physiology that is preventing the supplement from working the way it does in other people. A knowledgeable health care professional can evaluate these situations and find out exactly what is going on.

Q: Overall, what is the best way to approach exercise and sports competition?
A: When it comes to sports and exercise, most people want to excel. Some people are satisfied doing the best they can, while others always want to be number one and beat all their competitors every time. So it is possible to become obsessed with your sport, to become a fanatic and overdo it to the exclusion of everything else in your life, which is definitely not healthy.

If you are so competitive that your life is ruined if you don't win every time or if you aren't the best at whatever you are doing, that is not good. Having a healthy attitude toward exercise and sports means doing them in moderation, enjoying what you are doing, and being satisfied with a performance that is good for your individual capabilities.

For many dedicated athletes, a sports psychologist can be a good health care professional to consult. Some of them work on controlling the mind during competitions, which can help athletes to improve performance. They can also help you work on your attitude towards sports in general and, especially for those who are obsessed with competition, form a healthier perspective on the role of sports in your life.

Finally, stress reduction techniques can also be useful in improving performance. It is possible to get too worked up or anxious about competitions, which can impair your performance.

Physiologically, I think this kind of anxiety causes an imbalance in your autonomic nervous system. Research has shown that feelings of compassion boost the immune system and feelings of anger suppress it. So your emotions definitely affect your body and your ability to perform physically, including athletic performance.

Q: In summation, how does creatine supplementation fit into an individual's program of exercise and sports?
A: Creatine is a great supplement. It is highly effective for developing athletic strength and building muscle. But you also have to remember that creatine is only a supplement, and it cannot take the place of hard work—regular, consistent hard training sessions—plus a good diet, proper rest, and a healthy lifestyle.

When you combine creatine supplements with these other factors, the results can be astonishing. I've seen them in myself and in many of the patients I've worked with over the years. And you can see the change in just a few days. Creatine is a supplement with many different uses, and if you know what you're doing, you can really benefit from taking it.

Index

function of 93, 116, 164
Lou Gehrig's disease 56
magnesium 140–41
McArdle's disease 57
MedLine 192
mental function 152–53
mercury 77
methionine 25–27, 30, 173
minerals 162, 169–70
mitochondrial cytopathy 57
muscle mass (see also "crea-
	tine, muscle mass and")
	13, 22, 155
	gaining 14, 16, 21, 22,
		38–39, 46, 53, 69–70,
		105, 117, 125–127, 131,
		134–136, 148–49
	loss of 14, 21, 54, 59
muscle 38–43, 178–79
	building of 32–33, 43
	functioning of 36
	injuries to 42
	recovery after exercise and
		39–40
	storage of creatine in 27, 32
	types of 35–36
muscular dystrophy 10, 57
myasthenia gravis 57
nausea 107
nitric oxide 26
nutrient deficiencies 154
obesity 150
omega-3 fatty acids 166
olive oil 168–69
ornithine 137
	build-up of 46
osteoporosis 150

over-training 41, 181, 186
Parkinson's disease 10, 57–59,
	152, 172
phytochemicals 169–70
protein 25, 26, 28, 33, 37, 40,
	41, 138–39, 162–63
	egg as source of 164–65
	supplements 162–63
protein synthesis 33, 40, 43,
	70, 101, 164, 182, 185
pyruvate 137
rest 181–82
rhodiola 176–77
"roid rage" 128–29
sleep disorders 181
sports 13, 15–16, 33, 46–47,
	52, 63–74, 109, 112,
	121–22, 126, 143, 172,
	183
steroids 17, 21, 46–48, 72, 93,
	113, 121, 126–132
strength 13, 14, 20, 21–22,
	43, 53, 56–57, 61, 68,
	70, 85, 105, 149, 173,
	192, 195
stress reduction 182, 194
stretching 183
stroke 151
sugar, refined 161
supplements, general use of
	177, 193–94
taurine 97
testing, laboratory 184–89,
	193
testosterone 115, 126,
	130–134, 163, 185
thiourea 77

About the Authors

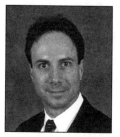

Dr. Joseph A. Debé is a 1986 graduate of the Southern California University of Health Sciences, from which he received his doctor of chiropractic degree. He is a Diplomate of the American Clinical Board of Nutrition, a Certified Clinical Nutritionist, and a Certified Dietitian-Nutritionist. Dr. Debé is also certified in sports injuries and physical fitness and practices at North Shore Fitness, a health club in Great Neck, New York. Dr. Debé has treated and counseled national and world champion athletes and has advised many on creatine supplementation. Dr. Debé is himself a former competitive weightlifter and has personally used creatine and enjoyed its many benefits. In addition to creatine, Dr. Debé has lectured and written extensively on a variety of health, fitness and nutrition topics. Many of his published articles are available on-line at www.drdebe.com.

Dr. Debé is a member of the American Academy of Anti-Aging Medicine, the International and American Associations of Clinical Nutritionists, and the Council on Nutrition of the American Chiropractic Association. His views regarding numerous health topics have appeared in a variety of media, including television, radio, video, newspapers, magazines and books.

Donna Caruso is a New York writer who specializes in health and nutrition topics. She is the author of *A Woman's Guide to Regaining Bladder Control.*

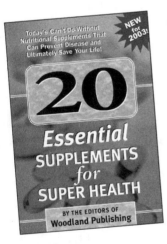
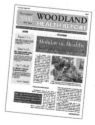